W9-BUF-970

52 SMALL CHANGES
FOR THE MIND

52
SMALL
CHANGES
FOR THE
MIND

BRETT BLUMENTHAL

**IMPROVE MEMORY · MINIMIZE STRESS
INCREASE PRODUCTIVITY · BOOST HAPPINESS**

CHRONICLE BOOKS
SAN FRANCISCO

Copyright © 2015 by Brett Blumenthal.
All rights reserved. No part of this book may be reproduced in
any form without written permission from the publisher.

Library of Congress Cataloging-in-Publication Data:

Blumenthal, Brett.
  52 small changes for the mind / Brett Blumenthal.
      pages cm
  ISBN 978-1-4521-3167-2
1. Mental health—Popular works. 2. Stress management.
3. Well-being. I. Title. II. Title: Fifty-two small changes for the mind.

  RA790.B5569 2015
  616.89—dc23

                          2014039167

Manufactured in China

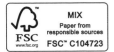

Designed by Amanda Sim

10 9 8 7 6 5

Chronicle Books LLC
680 Second Street
San Francisco, California 94107
www.chroniclebooks.com

TO ALEXANDER

My personal happy machine.
May your life bring you as much
happiness as you bring me.

CONTENTS

INTRODUCTION

SMALL CHANGES WORK. I know they do, because I've seen the results among many of my readers and other individuals who've abandoned the "change everything at once" approach for one that is geared toward making small changes over time. It makes sense: small changes are less overwhelming and more realistic, and they give us a sense of accomplishment more quickly. Regardless of the change a person wants to make, three things remain true: any major change actually requires many smaller changes; taking an all-or-nothing or extreme approach doesn't work; and small changes that we can manage and master feed our desire to succeed.

In my first small changes book—*52 Small Changes: One Year to a Happier, Healthier You*—I prescribe a small change each week for 52 weeks, so that by the end of the year readers are happier and healthier. The approach is holistic and addresses four dimensions of well-being: diet and nutrition, fitness and prevention, mental well-being, and green living. As I conducted research for *52 Small Changes* it became all too clear that I could have easily prescribed countless small changes within each of these categories.

When thinking through which topic of change I wanted to address next, I personally found the category of mental well-being (a.k.a. mental wellness or mental health) to be especially compelling. For many, maintaining good mental health is a bit elusive compared to maintaining good physical health. Understanding diet and nutrition or maintaining an exercise regimen is much more straightforward: you are either eating healthy or you aren't; you are either exercising or you're not. Moreover, when we are physically unhealthy, the symptoms are undeniable: we gain weight, we lose energy, we struggle with everyday tasks, and we feel lousy.

Mental well-being, on the other hand, has more gray area. For starters, most of us don't look at the whole picture when it comes to our mental well-being. We tend to focus on only one aspect: our happiness. While having good mental health most definitely means feeling happy and fulfilled, it also means that we can manage stress; we have a positive outlook on life; we can focus and concentrate when needed, so we are productive; and we can remember things easily. Some might even argue that a happy, healthy *mind* is the most important aspect of our overall health.

52 Small Changes for the Mind uses the approach of making small changes over the course of a year and applies it specifically to improving mental well-being. As with my first book, the changes prescribed are comprehensive, addressing multiple areas instrumental in achieving optimal mental health: stress management, concentration and productivity, memory and anti-aging, and of course, overall happiness and fulfillment.

Over the course of the next 52 weeks, I hope you'll find the changes to be fun and relatively easy to implement, and that you'll enjoy the process. The goal? By the end of the year, you should be able to manage stress, be more productive, remember more, ward off disease and aging, and feel happier and more fulfilled.

✦ ✦ ✦

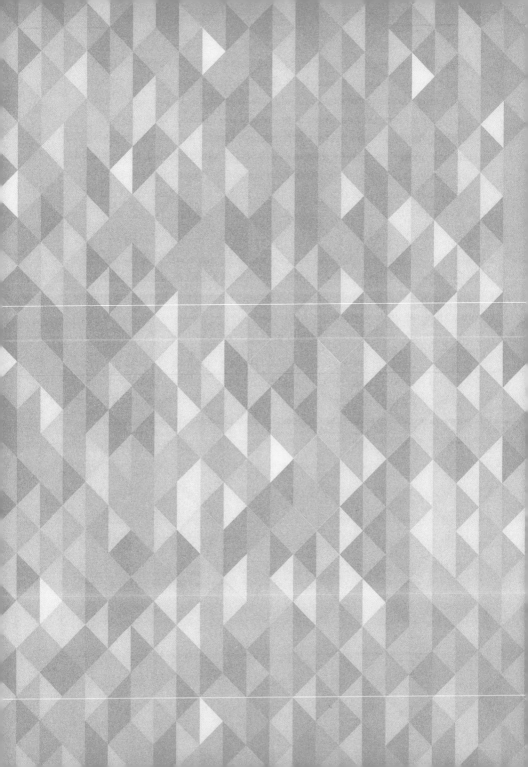

PART I

THE PROGRAM

HOW IT WORKS

THE *52 SMALL CHANGES FOR THE MIND* program is designed to encourage small yet meaningful changes that will ultimately lead to the big change of enjoying a happier, healthier mind. There are no gimmicks in here; just a clear, simple approach to help you be happier for the long term.

The idea is simple: make one small change per week for 52 weeks, and at the end of the year you'll feel less stressed and more productive, you'll remember more and ward off disease and aging, and you'll feel more fulfilled. This book is designed so that you can give yourself a year to make changes, which allows you to slowly integrate them over time, so they are more likely to stick for the long term.

Each change comes with an explanation of why it is important, as well as a "Path to Change," which provides tips and recommendations to help you successfully implement the change. With each week's success, you'll be inspired to move on to the next week's change so that within a year you'll have mastered all 52 changes.

Finally, to support you over the next 52 weeks, I've provided tools, worksheets, and other resources in Part III. I highly recommend you use these to stay motivated and on track throughout the program.

❖ ❖ ❖

A HOLISTIC APPROACH

THE PROGRAM OUTLINED in *52 Small Changes for the Mind* takes an integrated approach. At the beginning of each week's chapter, you'll see an icon signifying which of the four areas the change addresses. The changes have been organized so all areas are addressed throughout the

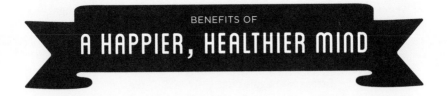

A HAPPIER, HEALTHIER MIND

INCORPORATING LIFESTYLE CHANGES to optimize your mental well-being will be very rewarding. When you make these changes, week by week, you can look forward to the following benefits:

+ **QUALITY OF LIFE.** These changes will help you reduce stress, anxiety, and worry, allowing you to live life to the fullest.

+ **STRESS AND COPING SKILLS.** You'll be better prepared to take on life's challenges and cope in a more productive and effective way. You'll feel more comfortable trying new things and taking risks.

+ **RELATIONSHIPS.** You'll connect on a deeper and more meaningful level with loved ones, enabling you to enjoy healthier and more rewarding relationships.

+ **INTELLECTUAL GROWTH.** You'll feel intellectually challenged, will develop greater creativity, and will be ready and willing to learn new things.

+ **PRODUCTIVITY.** You'll be able to concentrate and focus on tasks at hand, making you more productive both at work and in your personal life.

+ **OUTLOOK.** You will enjoy a happier, more positive outlook, which will extend into all areas of your life.

+ **YOUNG AT MIND.** You will take steps to become more youthful in mind and spirit, to remember and recollect things more easily, and to potentially ward off age-related mental decline and disease.

+ **SELF-ESTEEM.** When you are happy and feel good mentally, it translates into a healthy level of self-confidence and self-esteem.

52 weeks, rather than in sequential clusters. This will keep you engaged, interested, and motivated and allow you to comprehensively make progress. The icons are as follows:

 Stress Management

Concentration and Productivity

Memory and Anti-Aging

Happiness and Fulfillment

Every quarter, you'll find a helpful checklist of the changes you've made up until that point, so you can keep track of your progress and be sure to keep integrating them into your lifestyle.

✢ ✢ ✢

LIFE AFTER THE 52 WEEKS

THE GOAL IS that once you've completed the 52-week program you'll feel less stressed, have greater focus and concentration, have improved recall and memory, and feel all-around happier and more fulfilled than you do today.

Consistently maintaining all 52 changes, however, may not always be seamless and easy. There may be times when it's a bit challenging or your schedule makes it difficult. This is part of life, so don't let slipups discourage you. Life is a constant balancing act and requires us to make sacrifices. When you feel like you aren't on top of everything you could do for your mental health, remember: tomorrow is a new day. Approach each day with new motivation and resolve. In the end, integrating the prescribed changes *most* of the time is what's most important.

Revisit 52 *Small Changes for the Mind* often—it will continue to provide you with the basis for improved mental well-being so you can be at your best. And consider making the program a yearly project.

✣ ✣ ✣

GO YOUR OWN WAY

ALTHOUGH I'VE DESIGNED 52 *Small Changes for the Mind* to be followed over the course of a year and with a certain progression, it is ultimately your own personal journey. Use this program in whatever way works best for you. I do highly recommend you take at least a week to integrate each small change before moving on to a new one, but if you find one change really easy or you are already incorporating it into your lifestyle, feel free to move on to a different change. Additionally, if you don't want to use this book sequentially but prefer to go out of order, that is fine too. I would emphasize, however, that you should (1) take your time so the changes you make stick, and (2) no matter what timeline you use, be sure to incorporate all 52 changes into your life, as they are meant to work together in concert.

✣ ✣ ✣

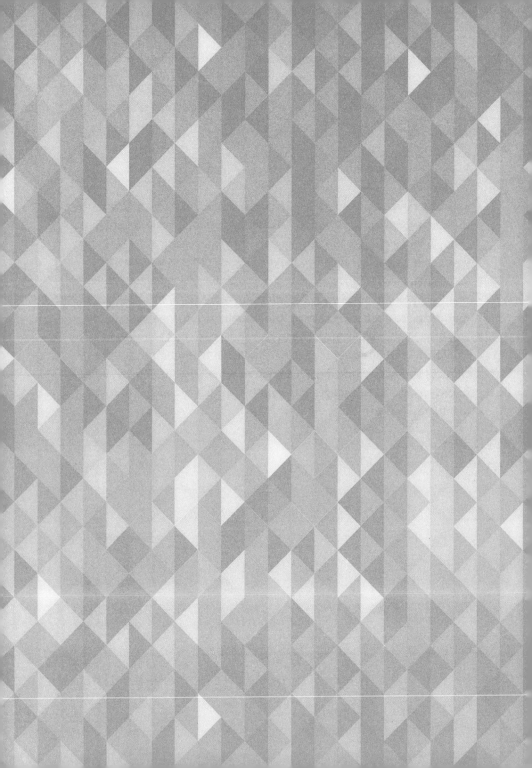

52 WEEKS OF HABITS

PUT PEN TO PAPER

WEEK 1

> The nicest part is being able to write down all my
> thoughts and feelings; otherwise, I might suffocate.
> —ANNE FRANK

ONE OF THE first and easiest changes to make is to start a personal journal. Journaling allows you to freely and openly express your deepest feelings without censorship or the interference or judgment of others. Journaling gives you an opportunity to be with your innermost thoughts, so you can think through situations and life, and explore them at a deeper, more meaningful level.

DID YOU KNOW?

The act of journaling dates as far back as the second century C.E., when the Roman emperor Marcus Aurelius wrote *To Myself*.

When we are confronted with difficult situations, journaling helps us sort through the issues so we are better equipped to see things more clearly, process and reflect on our reactions and thoughts, and problem-solve. When misunderstandings or disagreements arise with others, journaling helps us reflect on other people's perspectives and be more open to how they may be feeling or thinking. We become more intentional in our interpretations and better equipped to organize our thoughts so we can approach problems calmly and rationally. Journaling also encourages a free flow of thinking, which can tap into the more creative, intuitive right side of our brain to potentially reveal more innovative solutions.

Maintaining a journal encourages greater self-awareness and promotes a deeper connection with our emotions, even those that are difficult or painful. The more connected we are to our emotions and thoughts, the more prepared we are to experience growth and personal development. We are better equipped to identify our dreams, passions, and fears, and the things that need change. We also become more comfortable with who we are, which increases self-confidence and enables a clearer under-standing of relationships, situations, and needs so they can be better met. Further, written disclosure of emotions helps us learn lessons from our experiences, while staying in a positive and constructive frame of mind.

EMOTIONAL DISCLOSURE: A DRUG-FREE ANTIDEPRESSANT

In a 2008 study, outpatient psychotherapy clients saw significant reductions in anxiety and depressive symptoms, as well as greater overall progress in therapy when the client was asked to complete written emotional disclosure assignments, as compared with those who completed a writing assignment unrelated to emotional disclosure.[1]

Finally, journaling facilitates healthy stress management and increases happiness. The act of writing down feelings releases them out into the world so they don't stay bottled up; this leaves us calmer, happier, and more capable of moving past negativity. And when there is good in our life, journaling helps us to stop and take time to appreciate and savor the positive vibes we feel as well.

✢ ✢ ✢

THE PATH TO CHANGE
KEEP A JOURNAL

PUTTING PEN TO paper (or fingers to keyboard) is a therapeutic way of getting to the heart and soul of your innermost thoughts, feelings, and views on life and your experiences. Reap the benefits that journaling provides with some of these tips:

START WITH A GOAL Although it may feel forced in the beginning, journaling should be an activity that feels natural and easy. If you are new to the practice, set a goal for a certain length of time—say, ten minutes per day or every other day—so that you get into the habit of writing consistently. As you start writing on a regular basis, you should start to feel your emotions, feelings, and thoughts flow more freely, and you may very well surpass your initial goal.

LET IT FLOW There is no wrong way of journaling. This is completely about you, your world, and your own emotions, experiences, and thoughts. Try to let the words flow, and don't overthink what you are writing. There are no rules you need to follow. Don't get hung up on spelling, grammar, or even the length of your entry.

CHOOSE A TOPIC If you feel stuck or don't know what to write about, start with how you are feeling in that very moment. If it helps, you might consider choosing a theme for the day or week. Think about your relationships, your work, your dreams, and your fears. Engage your inner child in conversation, as children tend to speak their minds and thoughts more freely. Ask yourself questions about situations you're confronted with or experiences you've gone through.

KEEP IT PRIVATE If you kept a diary as a child or teenager, only to have it read by a parent, sibling, friend, or someone else, you may be a bit hesitant to make this change. As scarring as this past experience may have been, try to be open to reintroducing the habit into your life. There are many ways to ensure your privacy, and as an adult you have access to protections you didn't as a child. If you prefer journaling digitally, keep your journal as a file on your computer and have it password-protected. If you prefer to write in a paper journal, consider keeping it in a safe or under lock and key in a desk drawer.

JOURNAL IN MULTIMEDIA If you are creative or artistic, you might consider putting your journal into a multimedia format. You can create videos or voice recordings, sketch, paint, or use any other art medium you prefer.

JOURNAL YOUR CHANGES Because you will be going through many changes with 52 *Small Changes for the Mind*, consider keeping a separate journal or creating a special section specifically dedicated to tracking and recording your progress, your struggles, and your thoughts and feelings regarding the changes you're making. Transfer the activities from Part III: Tools and Resources, into your journal so everything can be found in one place.

✢ ✢ ✢

LET THE MUSIC PLAY

Music is a moral law. It gives soul to the universe,
wings to the mind, flight to the imagination, and
charm and gaiety to life and to everything.

—PLATO

MUSIC MAY HAVE existed since the beginning of life. Some of the first human-made musical instruments—flutes carved from bird bones and ivory—are said to date from thirty-five thousand to forty thousand years ago;[1] birds and sea mammals, among other species, have used melodies as a way to communicate with one another for as long as they've existed.

A universal language, music ignites passion and emotion in all of us. When a favorite song plays on the radio, our spirits immediately lift. A soothing song can relax and calm our nerves. A slow, somber melody may move us to be thoughtful, pensive, or sad. Music can inspire creativity and motivate us, and whether it triggers a subtle tap of our foot, a clap of our hands, or a dance involving our whole body, music physically moves us. Quite simply, music is transformational.

Studies have shown that music can start to have a positive impact on us as early as when we are first born (maybe even in the womb).[2] Dr. Van de Carr of Hayward, California, conducted research in the 1980s and found that prenatal stimulation between babies and parents, including playing music for the unborn fetus, produced significant differences in early speech, physical growth, parent-infant bonding, and success in breast-feeding, compared to those children and parents who didn't experience and provide such stimulation.[3] Once a child is born, listening to music can improve mood and reduce stress, enhance sleep patterns, promote good memory, and improve brain function and cognitive skills. Music can even help increase concentration and focus, as well as productivity and performance.

DID YOU KNOW?

Some research suggests that humpback whales compose their own music, using many of the same elements—such as rhythm, phraseology, and structure—that humans use.

Music has also been helpful in treating patients with dementia, anxiety, and other mental troubles, and has been instrumental in the treatment and recovery of surgical and cancer patients. One study found that music therapy increased comfort and relaxation and improved pain control for cancer patients; another found it improved quality of life.[4, 5]

Listening to music releases neurochemicals in the brain that directly affect our mental health. For example, the release of melatonin improves healthy sleep patterns, and dopamine helps to control the brain's reward and pleasure centers. When we listen to music that we don't like or find unsettling, however, we can activate the amygdala—the brain's fight-or-flight center—which in turn releases adrenaline.

Actively making music part of your life has a tremendously positive impact on mental well-being. Dr. Suzanne B. Hanser, coauthor of *Manage Your Stress and Pain through Music* and founding chair of the Music Therapy Department at Berklee College of Music, explains, "Almost every part of the brain is responsive to music in some way. The fact that [the brain has] such a multidimensional response [to music] is quite an amazing thing because there are few stimuli that can do that, and do it in real time. We change as we listen to music."

✢ ✢ ✢

THE PATH TO CHANGE
MAKE TIME FOR MUSIC EACH DAY

PUT MUSIC IN the forefront and give it a more significant place in your life. Some tips:

GET THE RIGHT EQUIPMENT There are many devices that make music appreciation easy and convenient.

Phone, iPod, or MP3 player Long gone are the days of bulky Walkmans or CD players; when you're out and about, play music on your phone, MP3 player, or other device, such as an iPod.

Headphones Invest in good headphones, especially if you are going to use them in loud or noisy places, such as airplanes, trains, and public areas. Choose noise-canceling headphones so you can keep music at an appropriate (and safe) decibel level, while blocking out distracting and less appealing sounds.

Home sound system For excellent sound quality, invest in excellent speakers. Choose the latest technologies to make integration with home devices as seamless and easy as possible.

GET ORGANIZED Load music into a digital library on your computer. Regardless of the application you use, your digital library will act as a central repository from which you can create playlists tailored to your mood. Download playlists and favorite songs onto mobile devices for listening on the go.

EXPAND YOUR TASTES Although you may have a favorite genre of music, seek out other genres as well. Different types of music can elicit different emotional responses and experiences. Further, our brains are activated differently by new music than by music with which we are familiar. For example, if you always listen to hip-hop or rock, you may tap into only one emotion or mental response. If, however, you listen to many other genres of music, such as jazz, classical, or opera, you will likely stimulate a wider variety of responses. Keep your repertoire fresh by regularly updating your library.

INTEGRATE MUSIC INTO YOUR LIFESTYLE Integrate music into your everyday activities at home and on the go:

Cooking Make cooking more festive and fun by listening to some upbeat tunes in genres such as Spanish guitar, swing, or jazz.

Housework and chores Make cleaning, laundry, and other household chores more fun and productive by pairing them with dance music.

Bring music outdoors Install a set of weatherproof speakers on your deck or in your yard so you can make music part of yard work, barbecuing, or family time outdoors.

Driving Go beyond the radio and get adapters for your MP3 player or mobile phone. You can also purchase satellite radio to access stations better suited to your tastes.

Walking the dog or commuting to work Make time pass more quickly by listening to your favorite music while walking Fido or riding the bus or train to work.

Exercising Choose high-energy music for workouts to increase their intensity. You may even burn a few extra calories from the extra energy boost.

Exercise	Electronica / Dance
Relaxation	Chill / Lounge
Focus	Movie Scores / Classical
Play	Today's Top 40 / Alternative
Creativity	New Age / Movie Scores
Entertaining	Jazz / Latin / Classical
Memory	'80s Pop

IN LIEU OF TV Watching television drains our energy, whereas listening to music ignites it and engages our brain. Replace a night of TV with a night of music. Search for new music, create new playlists, and share with friends, family, or loved ones.

MUSIC THERAPY   In *Manage Your Stress and Pain through Music*, Dr. Hanser dedicates a chapter to evaluating how music impacts individuals and their mood. Take the "Music and Mood Assessment" in Part III: Tools and Resources to evaluate different types of music and their emotional and psychological impact. Use the assessment to create playlists that best fit various activities and the emotional responses you want to stir during those activities.

IDENTIFY YOUR PERSONAL ANTHEMS   Movie soundtracks create a vibe that conveys what is happening during the movie. The soundtracks for the *Star Wars*, *Mission Impossible*, and James Bond movies are iconic. Create your own life soundtrack by choosing songs that speak to you on a deep and emotional level. Choose a theme song that ignites *your* personal aura. Do you want to feel powerful? Inspired? Sexy? Mysterious? Smart? Pick songs that make you feel the way you want, and play them when you need extra inspiration or personal motivation.

MAKE MUSIC Studies show that *making* music can provide even more benefit than listening alone. "When you engage in active music making, you use more parts of your brain, exercise more parts of your body, and have a much more robust experience, particularly if you are improvising, creating something new, or harmonizing a melody," explains Dr. Hanser. If you have already found a music-making outlet, be it singing or playing an instrument, try increasing your musical practice into your daily or weekly routine. If performing is new to you, take music lessons at a local music store or local school, sing in the shower, or try a fun evening out with friends doing karaoke.

HOST A MUSIC APPRECIATION PARTY Invite friends or family members over and ask them to bring a favorite album or song they think others don't know. Have guests discuss their selection, what they love about it, and how it makes them feel. Assign a theme to your parties so that over time you cover a variety of musical genres and push guests to expand their tastes.

✤ ✤ ✤

SHOW YOUR
PEARLY WHITES

Smile; it's free therapy.

—DOUGLAS HORTON

WHEN WE ARE especially stressed or feel as though everything is going wrong, it is easy to forget that smiling is an activity we can still enjoy, and one from which we can benefit. No matter the circumstances with which you are confronted—you're struggling with too many deadlines; you're contending with strains in your relationships; you've suffered a tragedy; or, pure and simple, you're having a bad day—there are always times when smiling doesn't come so easy. Yet making the extra effort is worth it.

Although the old adage "grin and bear it" may sound trite and virtually impossible when you are stressed or sad, studies show that a simple smile can be beneficial to our health, our mental state, and our overall outlook. For starters, smiling helps lower our heart rate and reduce stress levels. Tara Kraft and Sarah Pressman at the University of Kansas conducted a study that showed smiling through stressful tasks, even when forced and unnatural, resulted in lower heart rates during stress recovery among participants.[1]

Smiling also has a great influence on our mood. When we smile, we release endorphins, which travel down our spine sending feel-good messages throughout the rest of our body. These chemical neurotransmitters can reduce symptoms of both emotional and physical pain.

DID YOU KNOW?

Advances in ultrasound scanning have allowed doctors to see that babies start smiling in the womb, possibly as a reflex in preparation for life after birth.

The Facial Feedback Response Theory also suggests that the act of smiling makes us feel better and can improve our mood, even when we have to force it.[2] The more you smile, the more positive and happy you may feel. Similarly, the more you can reduce your negative expressions or frowning, the more you can reduce negative feelings or sadness. In a study conducted by Dr. Michael Lewis of Cardiff University in Wales, participants were given a Botox treatment for their frown muscles. Those patients who were unable to frown and express negative emotions facially had a significantly less negative mood than those who didn't receive the treatment.[3]

In addition to reduced stress and improved mood, your smile can often create happiness in others by eliciting smiles from those around you. This contagious response not only makes you happier, but it makes the other person happier as well. Smiling also has an extra social benefit: people find you more attractive and approachable. And, from an aging perspective, wrinkles that develop as a result of smiling are associated with a happier and more positive appearance.

Smiling is a holistic, natural "medicine." It helps us feel better, look better, and age better!

✢ ✢ ✢

THE PATH TO CHANGE
SMILE EVERY DAY,
AS MUCH AS POSSIBLE

MANY THINGS CAN get us to smile naturally, but smiling when we aren't used to it or are preoccupied with all of the have-tos that bombard us throughout the day can require some extra effort. Here are some ideas:

FAKE IT UNTIL YOU MAKE IT   Although you may not feel like smiling in the moment, try faking it. It may not feel genuine at the beginning, but at the very least it can produce the physical and mental benefits described here. Further, the more you practice smiling, the more naturally it will happen.

DID YOU KNOW?

In his TED Talk, "The Hidden Power of Smiling," Ron Gutman explains that on average, children smile approximately four hundred times a day, whereas only one-third of adults smile more than twenty times a day.[4]

SPEND TIME WITH CHILDREN AND PETS   Both children and pets tend to elicit natural smiles from us. Their playfulness, lack of inhibition, and general curiosity make them entertaining and funny. As a parent or a pet owner, enjoy as much time with your children and animals as you can. If you are childless and/or petless, look for ways to gain more exposure to children and animals. For instance, you might babysit or pet sit for friends, or volunteer at a school, animal shelter, or veterinarian clinic.

PRETEND YOU'RE A TV HOST   If you watch morning shows or entertainment television, you'll notice that many of the anchors and hosts have a continuous smile on their faces. Imagine you are a TV host and say everything with a smile (unless it is especially bad news, of course).

USE CUES Strategically place cues and reminders that will make you smile throughout the day. Some examples: displaying pictures of your children or your grandchildren, writing positive messages on sticky notes and posting them in key places around the house, setting cheerful computer alerts, or receiving daily inspirational quotes in your email in-box. Choose cues that work best for you and use them in a way that will bring a smile to your face. Dr. David Solly—a professor at University of the Rockies, a graduate institution specializing in social and behavioral sciences—suggests we create a "mental file" of those things that give us joy or peace, such as places we have visited and enjoyed, favorite hobbies and activities, or a personal victory. Scatter reminders of these throughout your home and workspace to keep you smiling as much as possible.

REFRAME NEGATIVE THOUGHTS TO POSITIVE Whenever you start to think negatively, smile and try to reframe the situation in a positive way. For instance, if you missed the bus on your way to work, you might smile and think about the possibility of meeting a new friend, running into an old friend, or having the opportunity to enjoy a little extra downtime before the hectic day ahead.

FIND A PERFECT DISTRACTION If you are feeling especially stressed or sad, find a funny or lighthearted distraction to enjoy. Maybe a website or book that has a "joke of the day" would be appropriate. Watch a funny video on YouTube or another website. Flip through some pictures of you having fun.

SMILE AT STRANGERS Depending on where you live, it may seem strange to smile at a complete stranger. Doing so, however, can boost confidence, make you happy, and, of course, rub off on the other person. Although it may feel awkward at first, the more you do it, the easier it will be.

STRENGTHEN YOUR SMILE   There are two types of smiles: those that are natural and genuine, resulting in a contraction of the muscles at the corner of the eyes (also known as the "Duchenne smile"), and those that are artificial. Most people can tell the difference between the two. Practice making your smile the biggest and most natural it can be, so when you flash your pearly whites, people know you mean it. Begin by looking in the mirror with a neutral face. Take note of how you look and the aura you present. Then, smile as if someone is about to take your picture. Say "cheese," if it helps. Again, note your aura and overall appearance. Finally, make your smile as big as possible, so much so that your eyes crinkle at the corners. Again, note your aura and how attractive you become as your smile gets bigger. Becoming aware of how you look with different facial expressions may help your smile grow over time.

UPGRADE TO LAUGHTER   Smiling has its benefits, but laughing is like smiling on steroids. Laughter eases anxiety and fear, improves our mood and outlook, and allows us to deal with difficult situations and disappointments more easily. Laughter helps draw attention away from negative emotions, such as anger, resentment, and worry, and allows us to instead focus on more positive emotions.

✤ ✤ ✤

BE A GOAL SETTER

If you want to live a happy life, tie it to a goal,
not to people or things.
—ALBERT EINSTEIN

NO MATTER YOUR age, goal setting is an extremely beneficial practice. Setting and pursuing goals gives life greater meaning and purpose, increases happiness, and gives structure to decision making and prioritizing.

Setting goals, big or small, promotes independent thinking—a key component to finding happiness. To truly see benefits, however, it is imperative you set goals that are authentic to you. Dr. Edwin Locke, professor of leadership and motivation (emeritus) of the School of Business at the University of Maryland, states, "People who choose their goals by copying other people's goals, will never be happy. When you do so, you don't have control over your life anymore." However, setting goals that are specific to your values, your interests, and what you personally want from life helps you think independently and freely and allows you to be the person you want to be. You gain a strong sense of responsibility and ownership of your successes and failures.

Setting goals helps improve self-esteem, which also contributes to happiness. Each time you achieve a goal and add it to your list of accomplishments, you prove you are capable of accomplishing what you set out to do, thereby boosting self-confidence and a deeper belief in yourself. Further, you become more aware of your strengths and all of the things you've mastered, helping to build your comfort in setting new goals. This confidence helps quash negative thinking, doubt, and fear, enabling a more positive outlook and a can-do attitude.

Setting goals can also be beneficial from an anti-aging perspective. As we get older, we can lose our sense of purpose, especially as our children leave the nest and we reach the age of retirement. Setting goals gives us a continued sense of purpose and pushes us beyond our comfort zone. Goals encourage us to be at our best; keep us challenged; help us develop new skills, thoughts, and opinions; and provide us with a natural way to keep learning. Staying in a growth mindset keeps us motivated and excited about life and our future and keeps our mind active, open, and flexible, all of which are important to warding off aging and maintaining memory.

Finally, setting goals allows us to prioritize our efforts. In order to achieve the goals we set, we must focus our activities, thoughts, and energy around them.

✛ ✛ ✛

THE PATH TO CHANGE
WORK TOWARD GOALS

WHEN YOU FEEL as though you are floundering or aren't quite sure where life is going, setting goals can help you get back on course. Here are some ways to set meaningful goals that inspire you and drive you toward greater happiness.

CHOOSE GOALS AUTHENTIC TO YOU   Avoid setting goals reflective of other people's beliefs or values. For instance, pursuing a medical career because your father and mother expected you to become a doctor is choosing a goal that essentially belongs to your parents. Instead, design your goals around what *you* want and your own values.

THINK BIG AND SMALL   Unfortunately, setting only big goals can feel overwhelming because they often take a lot more time and energy than smaller goals. So break down large goals into smaller, more digestible and manageable chunks (think 52 *small* changes). As you achieve each smaller goal, you'll feel inspired and motivated to continue with what is left to ultimately achieve the larger overall goal. Each smaller success will bring you a great sense of accomplishment and tremendous happiness. Maybe you want to spend more time with friends. Maybe you want to increase the time you spend on a favorite hobby. Or maybe you want to increase your time meditating or practicing yoga. All of these, although seemingly small, are valid and worthy goals. Sometimes smaller things in life bring us the greatest joy!

MAKE YOUR GOALS SMARTE   Many experts advise goals should be SMART—specific, measurable, actionable, relevant, and timely. However, I urge you to find an emotional connection to your goal so that your goal is SMARTE. With any goal you choose to set, big or small, you must be sure it is one you *want* to achieve. Use the SMARTE Goal Worksheet in Part III: Tools and Resources to guide you in making your goals.

DOCUMENT YOUR GOALS   Regardless of your goal's size, journaling your progress, your challenges, and how you overcome obstacles is a helpful exercise to keep you engaged in the process. Journaling keeps you accountable and provides you with a sense of responsibility for your successes and achievements. It also helps you take the goal more seriously. Merely thinking of a goal but not taking the extra step of writing it down can make it far too easy to not take it seriously—or to forget all about it.

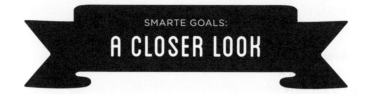

A CLOSER LOOK

WHEN SETTING GOALS, make them SMARTE. This will increase your chances of success.

SPECIFIC   Make goals specific and clear. Ask:

+ *What* do I want to accomplish?

+ *Why* is the goal important?

+ *Who* else do I need to help me accomplish the goal?

+ *Where* will I achieve the goal?

+ *Which* steps are necessary in order to accomplish the goal?

MEASURABLE   Measurable goals will allow you to evaluate progress and know whether you're headed in the right direction.

ACTIONABLE   Goals should be actionable. Ask:

+ Can I take action to work toward this goal?

+ Do I have the power to achieve it?

RELEVANT   Goals should be closely aligned with who you are and your values. Ask:

+ Is this goal meaningful to me?

+ Does it match my needs and values?

TIMELY   Give your goal a time frame for completion to keep you accountable and on track. Ask:

+ When do I want to accomplish this goal?

+ What can be accomplished in a few days? Weeks? Months? A year?

EMOTIONALLY DRIVEN   Goals should create a fire in your belly, a passion that continually inspires you to forge ahead. Ask:

+ Am I excited about this goal?

+ Do I feel inspired and motivated to accomplish it?

+ Can I keep motivation levels high all the way through to completion?

DID YOU KNOW?

In a study conducted by Dr. Gail Matthews of Dominican University, it was shown that individuals who documented their goals in writing and maintained a written log of progress were on average 33 percent more successful in accomplishing their goals than those who simply thought about their goals.[1]

MAKE YOURSELF ACCOUNTABLE When we share our goals with other people, we feel a greater sense of accountability. If, for instance, you want to lose weight and you know your friend or a family member also wants to lose weight, you might benefit from setting the goal together. You'll have each other to lean on for moral support and to keep each other motivated during the rough patches. Just be sure to choose people who are just as passionate and committed to the goal as you.

MAKE THE TIME Making time to achieve goals is a must for success. Build in the time you need so you can accomplish what you want, when you want. At the same time, be realistic about the timelines you set.

REWARD YOURSELF When you successfully complete a goal, always appreciate the work you put in and reward yourself for the effort you made.

DIVERSIFY Take a diversified approach to goal setting. Don't limit yourself to only one dimension, such as your career. The more dimensions of your life you address, the more well-rounded and accomplished you'll feel. Look for opportunities to set goals in your relationships, with your personal interests, at home, spiritually, intellectually, physically, and more. To help, make a goal matrix that includes the various areas in your life you want to address. Each time you achieve a goal, move to a different dimension in the matrix.

✦ ✦ ✦

MAKE LISTS

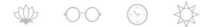

One of the secrets of getting more done is to make a
TO DO List every day, keep it visible, and use it as a
guide to action as you go through the day.

—JEAN DE LA FONTAINE

THIS WEEK'S CHANGE may seem overly simplistic, but making lists of
things you want (and need) to accomplish—in a day, a month, a year—
can be extremely helpful in eliminating stress, increasing productivity,
and even boosting happiness.

Trying to remember the endless number of tasks we need to get done can
be overwhelming, but when we take time to write things down, we
alleviate stress by removing the possibility of forgetting something and
having to pay the price later. According to Sonja Lyubomirsky, Ph.D.,
author of *The How of Happiness: A Scientific Approach to Getting the Life You
Want*, you can keep only seven to nine things in your working memory at
the same time. Making a list, however, allows you to free up brainpower
to analyze, prioritize, and even delegate tasks.[1]

Making and maintaining lists gives us a big-picture view of what needs
to get done, while giving organization and structure to a seemingly
disorganized mountain of tasks. We can easily prioritize our

responsibilities so we can avoid multitasking (in Week 6 you will learn how multitasking negatively impacts our productivity) and focus so we are most productive and efficient. And when we attach due dates to our tasks, we stay mindful of what is most pressing.

When we complete and cross or check off items on a list, we are rewarded with a huge sense of accomplishment. We feel successful, capable, and competent, all of which builds confidence and self-esteem, ultimately contributing to our happiness.

✧ ✧ ✧

THE PATH TO CHANGE
MAKING TO-DO LISTS

LISTS ACT AS an external hard drive for your memory and prompt you to stay focused. What has been overwhelming becomes manageable. However, if lists aren't used effectively, they can become a huge burden, adding more stress to our lives. Follow these basic rules:

CHOOSE YOUR FORMAT   If you are drawn to writing things down on paper, maintaining lists in a notebook or journal may be easiest for you. On the other hand, if you find technology more appealing and convenient, use your phone or other mobile device to maintain lists. Using technology instead of paper may provide additional benefits: you can sync lists with your calendar, create reminders, and easily update and revise them. There are also list-making/tracking apps, as well as online tools that sync with your phone and/or email account. That said, lists should make life easier, not more difficult. So choose whatever format most effectively fits with your personality and way of doing things.

KEEP IT SIMPLE AND MANAGEABLE   The more complicated you make lists, the less likely you will be to adhere to them and the more over-whelming they will feel. Overstuffing lists causes stress and confusion and may even sabotage your efforts to get things done. By the same token, too large a task can feel especially overwhelming and insurmountable. Keep to-do items simple, and instead of trying to tackle a very large task all at once, break it down into smaller tasks. As you make progress with each smaller task, you will stay motivated to keep forging ahead to complete the larger task.

ORGANIZE AROUND DEADLINES   Keep lists organized so you don't mix longer-term items with short-term items. Combining these on a list can result in more disorganization and clutter, impeding your ability to complete tasks and remain productive. Separate tasks that need to get done *that day* into one section, and have a separate section for items that can get done in the future. According to David Allen, author of *Getting Things Done: The Art of Stress-Free Productivity*, "If there's something on a daily to-do list that doesn't absolutely *have* to get done that day, it will dilute the emphasis on the things that truly *do*."[2] He asks you to write down everything you need to remember and to file it effectively. He explains that you should create a current task list that is relevant to today and the immediate future, and a "tickler file" of folders in which you organize reminders of things to do over the next month, as well as the next twelve months. For simplicity, David recommends that you create a task list for each day and a task list for the week and keep a "Future File" of longer-term items in a separate place. Revisit your Future File every week or two to stay mindful of those items and to assess if any of them should be moved to your current task list.

ORGANIZE AROUND PURPOSE   "Thing Lists" (such as shopping lists, invitee lists, and packing lists) definitely serve a purpose, as they too can help reduce the stress of forgetting items, but they should be kept separate from lists that require you to *do* something specific. Also, nothing on your list should be open-ended. For instance, "Think about the family vacation" is relatively open-ended and broad, whereas "Choose a destination for our family vacation" requires a specific result or decision. Similarly, "Work toward buying our dream home," although important, is open-ended and ongoing; "Deposit $500 in the home-to-be savings account" requires action and results in a completed task.

ORGANIZE LISTS AROUND AREAS OF YOUR LIFE   Keep personal to-do lists separate from work to-do lists. Doing so may help eliminate distractions. For instance, if you are using a list to meet a major deadline at work, seeing "Call vet for an appointment" on your list is going to distract and overwhelm you and diminish your focus.

PRIORITIZE   Every day, review each item on your list and give it a rating of A, B, or C, with A representing the most pressing or important tasks, B representing those next in line, and C representing those that can wait if need be. As you work through your tasks for the day, tackle them in order of importance.

CONQUER THE DISTASTEFUL   If you notice an item on your action list consistently popping up over and over, procrastination is likely at play. We often procrastinate for one of three reasons: (1) we don't really *need* to do something or it isn't very important, (2) the task is very difficult, or (3) it is essential, but we are so uninterested in the task we would rather deal with the potential consequences of not doing it than do what's required to be able to check it off our list. If a task is being put off for the first reason, then it shouldn't even be on the list in the first place. If the second reason applies, then it may be time to get help, delegate, or get input on how to complete the task. If, however, reason three is the barrier, consider enlisting the help of someone else to make it more tolerable. Or make a point of taking on that task first thing. Getting it done first means you are getting it out of the way so you can move on to more enjoyable tasks, and this will also give you a great sense of accomplishment.

REVIEW AND REWARD YOURSELF   At the end of each day, review your list to see how much you managed to accomplish. If you still have remaining items, create the next day's list beginning with those tasks. If you find you've completed tasks that were especially challenging or time-consuming, take a minute to revel in your achievement. Reward yourself with a break or something fun.

WHAT ISN'T ON YOUR LIST

Although we all need breaks during the day, there is a fine line between productive downtime and procrastination. If you suspect there is wasted time during your day, track how many hours you're spending on things not on your list. Take note of how much time you spend on the following activities: personal phone calls, surfing the Internet, social media, watching television, and unnecessary meetings at work. Once you understand how much time you spend on nonessential tasks, decide how much you are willing to give up to the greater good of productivity and how much downtime you really need. Then start scheduling breaks into your day so they are more intentional and have defined start and end times, to reduce wasted time.

REMAIN REALISTIC, FLEXIBLE, AND FORGIVING   There will always be days when the best-laid plans are hijacked by the unpredictable: you get stuck on the phone for hours; you get called into an unplanned meeting; your child is sick and requires a pickup from school; or you get a flat tire, making errands impossible. You can't predict every hiccup along the way, so remain flexible and forgiving when you don't accomplish all that you had hoped. Adhere to your prioritization, so if you can't get to everything, you can at least tackle the most crucial tasks for the day. And remember: tomorrow is a new day!

✤ ✤ ✤

BE A MONO-TASKER

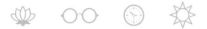

I think the one lesson I have learned is that there is no
substitute for paying attention.

—DIANE SAWYER

WE LIVE IN an age of multitasking. We email our colleagues while checking social media, chatting online, and talking on the phone. Although
multitasking may be benign in certain situations—such as watching
television while folding laundry—any activity requiring concentrated
focus, ensured safety, or meeting of deadlines is best done when we can
dedicate our full attention to the task.

Multitasking may seem like a more efficient way to get things done, but it
actually hinders our productivity, increases stress levels, and negatively
impacts our memory and our happiness. Although many who multitask
think they are good at it, research shows we are much more productive
when we focus on one single task at a time. In a 2010 study conducted by
James Watson at the University of Utah, participants performed two
tasks at once. A mere 2.5 percent of participants showed no decline in
performance, while for the other 97.5 percent, performance suffered.[1]
Moreover, habitual multitasking has been shown to have longer-term
effects. In a study conducted at Stanford University, it was found that

individuals who were considered heavy multitaskers had overall reduced abilities in filtering relevant information from irrelevant, diminished mental organization, and difficulty in switching between tasks.[2] And when it comes to multitasking when learning, studies show that the presence of distractions reduces our ability to learn.[3]

DID YOU KNOW?

Studies show that a person who is interrupted takes 50 percent longer to accomplish a task and makes up to 50 percent more errors.[4]

Multitasking also causes increased levels of stress, which can impact our memory. The constant stimulation we experience produces an adrenaline release (a stress response), which over time can damage cells that form new memories. As a result, constant high-stress multitasking can cause short-term memory loss.[5]

If multitasking is so bad for us, then why are we so eager to do it? Likely, because we receive a possible release of dopamine from the increased stimulation we get from multitasking, resulting in a temporary boost in happiness.[6] The constant distraction, however, can hurt our happiness level in the long term.

We receive a great amount of pleasure when we perform at our best and accomplish tasks well. But when we multitask, we sacrifice quality of work for quantity, so we experience both fatigue and disappointment with the lack of real results we produce. And the information overload we experience when we multitask can make it difficult for us to prioritize and make decisions, which can also diminish our overall happiness.

✦ ✦ ✦

THE PATH TO CHANGE
FOCUS ON ONE TASK AT A TIME

LEARNING TO MONO-TASK is beneficial to your productivity and ability to focus and reduce stress.

BUILD UP YOUR FOCUS TOLERANCE   If focusing on one task at a time is a challenge, time yourself. On day one, begin with twenty-minute intervals of focused time with five-minute breaks in between. On day two, increase your focus time to thirty minutes. The next day, forty minutes. Continue to extend the amount of time until you reach one-hour to two-hour spans of uninterrupted focused work.

MONITOR YOUR THOUGHTS   If your mind tends to wander when trying to focus, rein in thoughts and redirect them toward the task on which you are working. If, for instance, you are writing an email to a client and think, "I need to set up that conference call" or "I wonder if anyone has Liked my status on Facebook," stop and redirect your thoughts to what you are doing. If you can't get your mind off of other things, keep a running to-do list where you jot things down quickly and in the moment. This helps you to address the thought and redirect your attention back to the current task.

CAPITALIZE ON YOUR NATURAL RHYTHMS   Some of us can easily focus in the morning; others do so best later in the day. Evaluate when your peak focus times are, as well as the times you're most likely to be distracted. Plan important work during the times you know you'll be most able to focus, and more menial tasks for your less productive hours. For instance, if you know you're easily distracted around 3:00 p.m., do tasks at that time that don't require as much dedicated concentration, such as making phone calls, filing, organizing, or, if at home, laundry or cleaning.

CREATE THE OPTIMAL ENVIRONMENT   When concentration is essential, designate a space where you can retreat for your work. It should provide little to no distractions: no phones, computers (unless you need the computer to do your work), televisions, games, or gadgets, all of which are likely to sidetrack you. The space should be comfortable, but not so comfortable you become too relaxed or lethargic. The lighting in the space shouldn't be too bright or too dim, the temperature shouldn't be too cold or too hot, and the noise level should be appropriate.

Change of scenery Some find that working in the same environment all day, every day, hinders focus. If so, a change of environment can help you reengage in projects and tasks. Find a few different places where you find focused work easy to do.

Minimize clutter Keep your environment clear of extraneous papers, memos, and any other random items. Organize work areas so your sole focus can be on the task you need to complete.

DID YOU KNOW?

The United States Federal Government reports that in 2011, 3,331 people were killed, and an additional 387,000 people were injured, in car crashes involving a distracted driver.[7]

DON'T MULTITASK AND DRIVE Although car phones or hands-free devices are safer than talking on a cell phone you're holding with one hand, do your best to limit phone calls when driving. And most certainly never text while behind the wheel.

STREAMLINE COMPUTER TIME The computer has become ubiquitous with work. Unfortunately, it also encourages multitasking. Make computer work more focused with these tips:

Internet browser If you use the Internet for work, resist the urge to have multiple windows open. Instead, keep only one window and one tab open in a browser at a time.

Applications Keep your computer screen clear of clutter by using only the programs and applications you need at a time. Close any unnecessary documents and applications so they don't distract.

Alerts Computers distract with sounds and alerts. Every new "ding" breaks our concentration and requires refocus. Turn off your computer's sound and any alerts you don't need.

Schedule time for email and social media Social media and email can be a huge time waste. Instead of spending time on these activities throughout the day, designate specific times of the day for them. For instance, unless your work entails frequent essential communication by email, you might check and respond to your email twice a day, for a total of thirty minutes each—10:00 a.m. to 10:30 a.m. and 3:00 p.m. to 3:30 p. m.; and you might set up social media updates at 8:00 a.m. for ten minutes, and check in again at noon.

❖ ❖ ❖

FORGET THE JONESES

"Child," said the Lion, "I am telling you your story,
not hers. No one is told any story but their own."

—C. S. LEWIS FROM *THE HORSE AND HIS BOY*

COMPARING OURSELVES TO others starts at a young age. When we are
children, we compare ourselves with classmates, siblings, teammates,
and friends. As we get older, we find ourselves adding to the mix: comparisons with neighbors and colleagues, and, dare I say it, celebrities.
Whether we compare our grades, our looks, our income, our children, our
family, our possessions, or our perceived happiness, the practice often
leaves us feeling empty and unsatisfied.

Making comparisons can be beneficial in some instances, such as when
they inspire us to set new goals or be better people. But more often than
not, comparison robs us of joy, increases stress, and promotes dysfunctional behavior. It eats away at our self-worth and has the power to
undermine our accomplishments and damage our relationships. Comparing can cause resentment and jealousy, and it creates an unhealthy
level of competition between even the best of friends or closest of family
members. And, of course, when comparisons compel us to spend money
irresponsibly to "keep up with the Joneses," it can hurt us financially.

DID YOU KNOW?

In a 2005 study published in the *Quarterly Journal of Economics*, it was found that individuals reported lower levels of happiness when they learned their neighbors had higher earnings.[1]

Our need to compare comes from a belief that we aren't good enough as we are. These thoughts and feelings can cause a never-ending cycle of always wanting and looking for more, and never feeling satisfied with what we already have. Further, relying on comparisons to tell us we are okay prevents us from living in a genuine and authentic way. Instead, we rely on others to dictate how we feel, what we want, and how we live. In contrast, those who rely on *self*-approval don't need to compare because they know they are living in a way that is best for them, consistent with their values, and appropriate to their circumstances.

✧ ✧ ✧

THE PATH TO CHANGE
STOP COMPARING YOURSELF TO OTHERS

IF YOU'VE FALLEN victim to constant comparing, this change may feel especially challenging. Self-awareness and a little practice, however, can go a long way. And as you start to feel the benefits of stopping this behavior—increased happiness and self-esteem, improved relationships, and lower stress—you'll be more inclined to maintain a noncomparing or low-comparing attitude.

RAISE AWARENESS The habit of comparing can be deeply rooted; you may not even realize you do it. Build self-awareness around the behavior by staying on the lookout for comparing thoughts, such as thinking,

"I wish I were like . . ." or "I wish I had [fill in the blank] like . . ." or "I wish my spouse were more like . . ." These thoughts are often accompanied by bad feelings about yourself and lower self-worth.

ACKNOWLEDGE AND UNDERSTAND   If you notice yourself comparing, first stop and acknowledge the fact that you are doing it. Don't beat up on yourself for comparing. Instead, accept that you are doing it and ask yourself, "What is causing me to feel the need to compare?" Think about how it makes you feel and how it impacts you. Does it make you feel sad, or jealous or envious? Does it make you feel bad about yourself or your situation? Does it make you feel bitter toward the other person?

REFOCUS YOUR THOUGHTS   Many of us compare because we think or feel we are inferior. Shift your thinking from negative to positive by focusing on the good things in your life. Instead of thinking "I want" or "I wish," focus on the things for which you are grateful and thankful. Remind yourself that "more" doesn't always equate to happiness. Write down the things that make you happy and cause you joy. Count and appreciate the things you have, not the things that you lack.

MAKE CHOICES PREDICATED ON YOU   Comparing often leads us to want things that have very little to do with our own needs or preferences. Predicate your choices in life on what you deeply want, not what the external world makes you *think* you want. If, for instance, you want to lose ten pounds, do so because *you* want to, not because you are concerned with what others think. Or if you want to buy a new car, do so because *you* genuinely like and want that car, not because your neighbor or best friend has the same one and you are trying to fit in or keep up. Make decisions that satisfy you deeply, rather than to impress others.

BUILD SELF-ESTEEM AND SELF-APPROVAL   A big part of the reason we compare is that we don't accept ourselves for who we are. The more you can love and embrace yourself, the more you will feel at peace and content with the life you have. A few things to work on:

Know your values The more you know your values and understand what is truly important to you as an individual, the less likely you'll be to compare. Your values will dictate your choices and decisions and will allow you to put less emphasis on what everyone else has or is doing. Spend some time thinking about what is most important to you (such as family, money, gratitude, happiness, authenticity, honesty) and write down the five things in life you value most.

Celebrate your uniqueness Every one of us is unique, and this should be celebrated! If we were all the same, the world would be quite a boring place. When you feel the urge to compare, remind yourself that your uniqueness is what makes you special. To go one step further, you can purposely _choose_ to be different. Taking the less popular route makes it okay to not be like everyone else or have what everyone else has. You are making a choice to be different, so you are purposefully removing the potential for comparison.

Observe your strengths When you start to feel negatively about what you lack, think about all of the amazing qualities you have. Maybe you are generous and kind. Maybe you are especially skilled at leading. Maybe you are a talented singer. Remind yourself of the things you are exceptional at and how likely it is that others wish they had _your_ talents.

REALIZE THERE'S MORE THAN MEETS THE EYE   It is human nature to put our best foot forward for others. Although things may look great on the surface, however, there's always more to a situation or a person than meets the eye. For instance, maybe a couple appears to have the perfect marriage, but they constantly fight in private. Or maybe a friend has a beautiful house and a fancy car and goes on exotic vacations, but deep down she is unhappy and lonely. Realize that when it comes to others, you see only a small piece of the puzzle.

FOCUS ON NONMATERIAL THINGS   Comparing often focuses on the materialistic or quantifiable things people have instead of the quality. Cars, clothes, houses, income, and the like are all quantifiable. Yet family, health, friends, and our life experiences make life much richer. Spend more time enjoying the nonmaterial side of things and your personal journey through life instead of on the "things" you have or don't have.

BE LESS CRITICAL OF OTHERS   Just as it is unhealthy and unproductive to compare with others, it is also unhealthy to criticize or judge others to make yourself feel better. Try to support others in being unique and celebrate their differences, just as you should celebrate yours.

AVOID ACTIVITIES THAT CAUSE COMPARING   Some activities lend themselves to drawing comparisons more than others. For instance, reading tabloids and watching certain types of television shows keep us in a superficial, comparing mindset. And, of course, gossiping is the quintessential comparing activity. Reduce these types of activities in your life, and instead focus on those that are more meaningful and bring out your most positive qualities.

DEAL WITH ENVY   If you constantly feel jealous or envious of others, identify why you are envious. Look past the superficial and get to the heart of what is really driving those feelings. Is it insecurity? Is it your job and salary? Is it a lack of strong relationships in your own life? Try to detach your emotion from the situation. Objectively celebrate the other person, and think about how you can bring qualities into your own life that address your envy. Use the person as inspiration or as a role model instead of as someone with whom to compete.

✢ ✢ ✢

MEDITATE

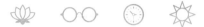

The present moment is filled with joy and happiness.
If you are attentive, you will see it.

—THICH NHAT HANH

ALTHOUGH THE TERM "meditation" may conjure up images of monks in a remote Tibetan monastery vocalizing a resounding "om," the practice of meditation can be very simple and accessible and can be done virtually anywhere at any time. Meditation has existed for thousands of years and provides tremendous benefit to our well-being, both mentally and physically. Those who practice meditation experience a sense of calm, peace, and balance, even well after the meditation session is over.

Thanks to research in the field of mindfulness and the popularity of yoga, meditation has become widespread in the last several decades. Those who practice can clear away the clutter in their minds and bring clarity and focus into their lives. They gain new perspective, enjoy a more positive outlook, manage stress better, and achieve a deeper level of self-awareness.

Meditation can also have a positive and lasting impact on our memory and learning processes. Studies show that meditating on a habitual basis can lead to increased gray matter in the hippocampus and other brain structures associated with learning and memory, while decreasing the density of gray matter in the amygdala, which correlates with reduced stress.[1] Meditation also allows us to calm the mind and clear out distracting thoughts, which heightens our ability to focus and concentrate. In a study conducted at the University of Washington, participants who were part of a meditation program saw a decrease in task-switching and were able to focus on tasks for longer periods of time. They were also able to recall details of the work they did more accurately compared to those who did not participate in a meditation program.[2]

Finally, meditation asks that we remain in the present and release judgment, past hurts, and negative thoughts and experiences, so we can find inner peace and achieve greater positivity and happiness.

✢ ✢ ✢

THE PATH TO CHANGE
MEDITATE TWENTY MINUTES PER DAY

THERE ARE MANY ways to meditate and many forms of meditation from which to choose. If you are new to the practice, however, it is best to start simple. To begin your practice:

MAKE A COMMITMENT   To really reap the benefits of meditation, you should commit to making it a daily practice. If you are completely new to meditation, you may want to start with a five-minute block of time, working your way up to about twenty minutes per day over a few weeks or even a few months.

PICK A PLACE   Find a place conducive to quiet serenity. This could be outside at a park, in a quiet room or nook in your home, or even at the beach. It doesn't matter where you choose, as long as you can sit without interruption for a block of time—ideally up to twenty minutes. Make sure there is as little noise as possible. Some people prefer to listen to music, but if you do, choose very soft, rhythmic music, and avoid tunes with lots of words or heavy beats, which can be distracting.

CHOOSE A TIME   Choose a time of day when you are most likely to remain undistracted or undisturbed and when you can dedicate a block of time. For many, early morning or later at night is a good time. You should also use a timer to let you know when you've completed your practice.

GET INTO POSITION   During meditation, comfort is key. Your clothing and even the way you sit should be very comfortable. Avoid binding or restrictive clothing and clothing that makes you too hot or not warm enough. Although it is traditional to sit Indian style with your hands resting on your knees or in your lap during meditation, it is most important that you sit in a comfortable erect posture that requires you to support your head with your neck, as opposed to by a headrest on a chair or couch. This erect posture keeps you from falling asleep. Some common positions include sitting on a pillow on the floor or in a firm chair. Rest your hands in your lap or on your knees. Finally, lightly close your eyes. Although it is possible to meditate with your eyes open, it is easier to avoid distractions when your eyes are closed.

SET AN INTENTION FOR YOUR PRACTICE   Start your meditation with a reminder of why you want to meditate. Some ideas: you want to feel relaxed and let go of stress, you want to let go of anger or resentment, you want to clear your mind, or maybe you simply want to be more mindful and in the present moment.

FOCUS   Maintaining focused attention throughout your meditation is key. The goal is to avoid thoughts about your life or problems. Some things to focus on:

Your breath Focusing on your breath is one of the most common ways to meditate. And it is great for beginners because it is a natural function. Your breath should come from deep within your abdomen (as your diaphragm rises and falls) and not your chest (that is, your chest should barely rise, while your abdomen expands and contracts with each breath). As you breathe, concentrate on feeling and listening as you inhale and exhale. Follow the breath as it enters your nose, your throat, and your lungs. When you exhale, be mindful of the breath as it leaves each of these areas of your body. Here are couple of ways to concentrate on your breath:

> ✤ FIVE COUNT _As you inhale, count slowly to five. Hold for a second, and then exhale for a count of five. Repeat this process until your timer signals you are done with your session._

> ✤ COUNT PER BREATH _Count each inhalation and each exhalation. On the first inhalation, count one. On the exhalation, count two. Count three on the next inhalation and four on the next exhalation. Continue counting until you reach ten. When you get to ten, restart your counting from one on your inhalation. Continue this process until your timer signals you are done with your session._

A mantra Quietly recite a mantra: a specific word or several words that bring you a sense of peace and serenity. Your breathing should remain deep and rhythmic as you repeat your mantra. Continue repeating the mantra for the full time of your meditation.

Guided meditation Many athletes use guided meditation as a way to prepare for a race. Essentially, you focus and direct your imagination toward a conscious goal. For instance, a marathoner might imagine himself running through the racecourse from the start to the finish line, prior to running the race.

An object If you are comfortable meditating with your eyes open, you can focus on an icon or object that has meaning to you. Some ideas: a statue of the Buddha, a flower, a garden, the ocean, or a cross. If a desirable object isn't in front of you, you can also close your eyes and use your imagination to visualize an object. Keep your attention fixed on the object as you breathe deeply.

<u>Your body</u> Conduct a mental body scan, focusing your attention on various parts of your body. Be mindful of the sensations you feel: pain, relaxation, tension, temperature, or numbness. You may also want to try to tense and then fully relax different parts of your body. For instance, start with tensing your fingers and then relaxing them. Move to your hands, your arms, your shoulders, and so on, until you address all areas of your body. Combine this, again, with deep breathing.

THE WANDERING MIND

Throughout your meditation, you may find your mind wanders. If this happens, take note of your thoughts briefly, and then return your focus to your breath, your mantra, or whatever else you are focusing on during your meditation. Whatever you do, however, do not go into a place of judgment or criticism. It is common for the mind and attention to wander during meditation. Be open and loving to yourself during your practice.

BUILD UP TIME   Aim to meditate for five minutes at the beginning of your practice. Do so for seven days, and then increase your time to ten minutes. When you can meditate consistently for ten minutes on days seven through fourteen, increase your time to fifteen minutes. When you can meditate for fifteen minutes on days fourteen through twenty-one, then increase it to twenty minutes.

LEARN A TECHNIQUE   The meditation techniques discussed here are very simple and a great way to begin. There are many other forms of meditation one can practice, each providing unique benefits and appealing to different types of individuals. Some more popular types include Transcendental Meditation (TM), Mindfulness Meditation, Kundalini, Qi Gong, and Tai Chi. Search online to learn about the various types of meditation you can practice and to find meditation centers in your area that may give classes on the specific types that interest you most.

INCREASE TO TWO TIMES PER DAY Once you are able to meditate for a twenty-minute block each day, consider increasing your meditation ritual to twice daily. Many experts state that twenty minutes twice daily is ideal. What's most important, however, is the quality of your meditation. Be sure the twenty minutes you dedicate to your practice brings you the mindfulness you seek.

GO ON A RETREAT There are many meditation centers and wellness spas that provide weeklong or weekend retreats for individuals interested in intensifying or strengthening their meditation practice. Consider taking a yearly retreat that allows you to learn and expand your practice.

✤ ✤ ✤

KICK INDECISION

Twenty years from now you will be more
disappointed by the things that you didn't do
than by the ones you did do.
—H. JACKSON BROWN, JR.

WE ARE FACED with decisions every day. Committing to a simple choice, however, may not be as easy as we'd like. Indecision often stems from fear, driven by concern that we will make the "wrong" decision. We suffer from a need for certainty, a need for the best results, and maybe even a need to be right. In most cases, however, there may not be a "right" decision—just different options. Further, many decisions can be perfectly good ones, as long as they move us in a direction. As a result, agonizing over the "correct" decision can cause a lot of wasted time, anxiety, and stress, and in some cases, diminished happiness and joy.

When we look at decisions through a lens of right or wrong, we limit ourselves from experiencing the unexpected. Although keeping our options open may seem optimal, it can keep us stagnant. In truth, as much as you'd think people regret making the wrong decision, regret is often a result of *lack of action*. Even a perceived *wrong* decision can bring about better results than no decision at all.

❖ ❖ ❖

THE PATH TO CHANGE
BECOME A DECISION MAKER

IF YOU FIND that making decisions, big and small, sends you into a state of paralysis, try the following:

PRIORITIZE AROUND YOUR VALUES When facing decisions that impact your life, be especially mindful of your core values and what is important to you. Prioritizing based on *your* principles, as opposed to those of others, will allow you to make decisions more easily, based on what is in your best interest.

TRUST YOUR INTUITION Indecision can be driven by a lack of self-confidence and a belief that you are incapable of making decisions for yourself. It is important to trust your intuition and believe in yourself to take an appropriate course of action. Realize you have the power to create the life you want and to make choices that are best for you.

REJECT THE NOTION OF PERFECTION Looking for a perfect outcome can easily keep us stuck in an indecisive place. Remind yourself there is no such thing as perfect, right or wrong, or good or bad. Further, accept that things can be less than perfect and still be great. All choices can work. Not choosing, however, won't work. Making *any* decision provides you with benefits: you move in a direction, you learn more about yourself, and if the results of your decision don't turn out as you had hoped, you can always change course.

OUTSOURCE WHEN NECESSARY Although decisions should be predicated on your own goals and needs, it can be helpful to get an outside opinion from someone who knows you well. This especially holds true when making decisions about something of which you know very little. For instance, if you are trying to decide what kind of smartphone you want to buy but you find new technology overwhelming, ask your tech-geek friend or relative for a concise breakdown in layperson's terms of your various options and what would be the best fit for you.

DID YOU KNOW?

In a 2000 study conducted by Sheena Iyengar, Ph.D., a management professor at Columbia University Business School, and Mark Lepper, Ph.D., a psychology professor at Stanford University, it was found that although participants showed interest in having more choices, they were ten times more likely to make a choice if given limited options. Further, those who had a limited number of options reported greater satisfaction with their final selection.[1]

STREAMLINE OPTIONS Too many choices can contribute to indecision. If you are confronted with too many options, take control by creating limitations. For instance, if you have a difficult time deciding what you want to order when you go out to lunch, limit yourself to a specific part of the menu from which you will make a selection (say, sandwiches, salads, or pizza). Or take it one step further and limit yourself to only two or three options from the menu.

SET A TIME LIMIT Don't let decisions drag on for hours, days, even weeks on end. Give yourself an appropriate time limit so the indecision can go on for only so long. If you are in the market for a new mattress, limit yourself to one afternoon to make that choice. Or if you are deciding on what to wear for a night out on the town, limit the decision process to ten minutes.

SET PARAMETERS Before making a decision, select what parameters or prerequisites will guide you during the process. For instance, if you are looking to join a new gym, maybe atmosphere and quality of equipment are more important to you than the classes they offer or the cost. When making your selection, measure the choices against your biggest priorities to quickly eliminate those that don't meet them.

BECOME (A LITTLE) PREDICTABLE   Eliminate indecision from the day-to-day by becoming a little predictable. For instance, if you are satisfied with certain products or brands, stick with them. If the coffee menu at the local coffee house overwhelms you every morning, choose a drink and stick with it each day.

HAVE A CONTINGENCY PLAN   If you fear making a bad decision, imagine the worst-case scenario that could result. Next, determine an appropriate course of action if that scenario were to occur. We are more prone to play out unrealistic negative scenarios in our head rather than positive ones, yet the worst-case scenario rarely happens. Putting an action plan in place in case something needs to be changed, however, can reduce stress from the seemingly unknown and allow you to feel more comfortable with the decision you do make.

DEAL WITH DISAPPOINTMENT   If you ever feel as though a decision you made wasn't the best or the results were disappointing, don't let it overcome you. Instead, maintain a positive attitude and look for opportunities to learn from the situation so you are better prepared to make decisions in the future. Accept the outcome, learn from it, and move on.

✤ ✤ ✤

SIP GREEN TEA

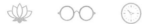

There is something in the nature of tea that leads us
into a world of quiet contemplation of life.

—LIN YUTANG

GREEN TEA HAS been imbibed by Asian cultures for centuries. Recently it
has been gaining popularity in Western civilization, and for good reason:
green tea has amazing benefits for mind, body, and spirit.

Due to its numerous phytochemicals, green tea is a powerhouse for
anti-aging and has been linked to a diminished risk of neurodegenerative
diseases, such as Alzheimer's and Parkinson's.[1] Research has shown that
the polyphenols in green tea, also known as epigallocatechin-3-gallate
(EGCG), can enhance neurogenesis of the hippocampus, which is important to learning and memory.[2] One of the tannins found in green tea—
gallotannin—helps prevent brain damage after strokes and other brain
injuries.[3] In a study of one thousand Japanese people ages seventy and
older, participants who had a higher consumption of green tea had lower
prevalence of cognitive impairment.[4]

Green tea has also been shown to provide stress relief. In a study out of
Japan, it was found that green tea consumption was inversely associated

with psychological distress.[5] Further, the polyphenols found in green tea have the power to raise levels of dopamine, a mood-boosting compound. In fact, research shows drinking green tea can have a positive effect in those who suffer from symptoms of depression.[6]

And if you are looking for a boost in concentration, focus, and productivity, green tea could be the perfect fix. Green tea has caffeine, a known stimulant, but in much lower doses than a typical cup of coffee. As a result, those who enjoy it don't suffer from the typical jitters that can occur when drinking too much coffee. The real magic in green tea, however, is that it uniquely contains the amino acid L-theanine. L-theanine has anti-anxiety effects and has been linked with enhanced mental alertness and attention.[7] The combination of caffeine and L-theanine makes green tea especially effective in boosting brain function.[8, 9]

✢ ✢ ✢

THE PATH TO CHANGE
CHOOSE GREEN TEA OVER COFFEE

GREEN TEA CAN be an easy add to your daily diet. Here are some tips to make it seamless:

HOW MUCH?   Although drinking some green tea is better than not drinking it at all, ideally you should aim for a minimum of two to three cups per day. In a study out of Japan, those who drank at least two cups daily were 54 percent less likely to exhibit cognitive impairment.[10]

MAKE A SWITCH   If you are a regular coffee drinker, trade in your cup of joe for a cup of green tea. If giving up coffee in the morning sounds painful, remember that green tea offers the benefits of caffeine without the jitters. Moreover, as it enhances focus and concentration, it is the perfect beverage to kick-start your workday.

ENJOY THROUGHOUT THE DAY   Typical brewed coffee contains approximately 95 mg to 200 mg of caffeine per 8 ounces. Green tea, however, contains only 24 mg to 40 mg of caffeine per 8 ounces. So you can enjoy more cups of green tea without the worry of overdoing your caffeine intake. If, however, you are sensitive to caffeine, avoid drinking green tea after 2 p.m. so as to not disrupt your sleep patterns.

DID YOU KNOW?

In a study conducted by David Weiss of the University of Colorado at Colorado Springs, it was found that the EGCG levels in matcha green tea (a finely ground powdered green tea) were 137 times greater than that found in typical China Green Tips green tea and three times greater than the highest documented value of other green teas.[11]

BE PICKY ABOUT DECAF   If you would prefer to drink decaffeinated green tea, it pays to be picky about which decaffeinated tea you purchase. There are two processes used to decaffeinate tea: (1) ethyl acetate and (2) carbon dioxide (CO2). The ethyl acetate process is a chemical process that strips the tea of some of its benefits and leaves solvent residue on the tea leaves. The carbon dioxide method, on the other hand, uses carbon dioxide and water to remove the caffeine, leaving the tea's polyphenols and catechins intact. Many manufacturers don't provide information about the process of decaffeination they use, and if a label says "naturally decaffeinated" it doesn't necessarily mean that ethyl acetate wasn't used. As a result, consider decaffeinating tea on your own. Simply steep tea for about forty-five seconds, then discard the liquid and add more hot water to steep a second time. Approximately 80 percent of the caffeine is released in the first minute of steeping, so you will remove most of the caffeine this way.

TRY MATCHA Matcha is a finely milled green tea made from the whole tea leaf. Unlike drinking traditional green tea, drinking matcha means you ingest the tea leaves, not just the water brewed from the leaves. Proponents claim you get many more benefits from matcha over regular green tea, including a dose of fiber. Matcha tea can be made traditionally by whisking the fine powder into hot water and then drinking it before the powder settles. You can also use matcha for lattes, smoothies, and even homemade green tea ice cream.

SPICES, HERBS, OR FLOWERS, OH MY! Green tea's flavor may not be your cup of tea (pardon the pun). If you aren't a fan of green tea's basic flavor, add some flavor with spices, herbs, or flowers. Some traditional additions include jasmine and lemongrass. Experiment with your own flavors. Some to try include cinnamon, rose petals, mint, or even citrus, such as tangerine or orange.

SWEETEN WITH ORGANIC RAW HONEY Although it is best to keep green tea unsweetened, if you need a bit of a sweeter taste, opt for organic raw honey instead of plain sugar. Unlike sugar, which provides no health benefits at all, honey delivers an extra boost of antioxidants. Because processing of honey strips away its antioxidants and other nutrients, choose raw, unprocessed honey. And of course, choosing organic means the bees aren't subjected to chemicals or pesticides.

✢ ✢ ✢

SEE THE BEST IN OTHERS

> Treat people as if they were what they
> ought to be, and you help them to become
> what they are capable of being.
>
> —JOHANN WOLFGANG VON GOETHE

WHETHER WE HAVE suffered personal offenses, watched too much crime on the news, or read too much drama in the tabloids, we have good reason to doubt the intentions of others. Unfortunately, this type of thinking not only impacts how we view other people, but also can impact our happiness and how we view ourselves. Finding the good in others, even when difficult, can prove to be beneficial: the more positives you see in others, the more you can see the positive in yourself. This boosts self-esteem and self-confidence, both of which are instrumental to success and happiness.

We are predisposed to think negatively about our fellow man. We have what's called a "negativity bias," which causes us to give more focus and more weight to negative experiences, thoughts, and information than we do to those that are positive.[1] Because of our negativity bias, we're more likely to notice the bad than the good in others. We are more likely to expect the worst. And we are more likely to be annoyed by someone's idiosyncrasies than we are to appreciate his or her good qualities. We want to be recognized for our positive qualities, our best traits, and our full potential. When we are critical and annoyed by everyone around us, it makes us less trusting, less generous, less open, and all-around less positive. In turn, we send a negative message to others, causing them to think we lack good in ourselves. Yet ironically, we want others to see past our own mistakes, missteps, and faults.

OUR EXPECTATIONS INFLUENCE OTHERS

Our expectations of others and our behavior can directly influence how others see themselves and their potential for success. Researchers found that when elementary school teachers expected enhanced performance from students, they tended to show enhanced performance.[2]

Essentially, people act in accordance with how they are treated. When you expect the worst in others, they tend to fulfill those expectations. When you think positively, people tend to act more positively. When we can overcome our negativity bias and see the good in others, it reaps amazing results. Others receive positive feelings of trust, respect, and safety, making them more inclined to feel the same toward us, and as a result, more drawn toward us. And when both sides can be more positive, it tends to bring out the best in all of us, and this quickly snowballs into making us feel happier, more confident, more loving, and generally like we are better people.

✢ ✢ ✢

THE PATH TO CHANGE
FOCUS ON OTHERS' POSITIVE QUALITIES

SEEING THE BEST in others requires an open heart and open mind. Some things to consider:

BE GENEROUS We all have good in us. Search for it in others, as well as in yourself. Take the time to know people and focus on their abilities, strengths, and positive characteristics. Try to be forgiving, nonjudgmental, unprejudiced, kind, open, honest, and accepting. This is important in connecting with others and the greater world around you. Be open to new individuals and relationships. Be helpful to those in need. Compliment people. And when you speak to others, be encouraging. Use phrases like "I trust you" and "I know you can do this."

AVOID GENERALIZATIONS Generalizations are usually inaccurate and hurtful. Remember that each person is an individual, with a unique personality, characteristics, and strengths. Don't assume that because someone is of a specific age, gender, cultural or ethnic group, religion, or economic status, you know who she is or what her capabilities are. Also, avoid using a person's past behavior as a generalization for all future behaviors. Understand we all have bad days (and years!), and those instances shouldn't define us as individuals. Just as you would hope others forgive your less than stellar moments, it is important to forgive those of others as well.

BE REALISTIC Although having high expectations of others can positively influence their behavior, holding people to too high a standard, expecting perfection, or having unrealistic expectations can backfire. Avoid expecting others to be perfect at all times.

BE A DETECTIVE When we think the worst of people, it is often because we rush to conclusions. Take the time to clearly understand situations and people's circumstances. Be open-minded, look for the good, and try to see people's actions as well-intentioned. When behaviors seem especially bad, try to assume there are valid underlying reasons. Maybe a driver honks on the road because he is rushing to get to the airport for a flight for which he is late. Maybe someone leaves a bad tip because she made a calculation mistake. Even when behavior is seemingly inexcusable, try to understand or imagine that it is for a logical reason.

ADDRESS YOUR INNER CRITIC When we have difficulty seeing good in others, it is because we have trouble seeing the good in ourselves. It can also be a result of having been raised or surrounded by critical people. Think about the source of your inner critic. Is it your own voice, really? Or is it a voice you've acquired over time because of the people you know? Identify the root cause of your critical thoughts so you can quiet them over time.

SHOW IT Let your body language speak to "seeing the best" in others. Look them in the eye to convey trust and respect. Smile to exude comfort and openness. These simple gestures show others that you think positively about them, see the good in them, and enjoy connecting with them.

✢ ✢ ✢

READ FOR PLEASURE

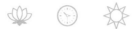

I have never known any distress that an
hour's reading did not relieve.

—CHARLES DE MONTESQUIEU

UP UNTIL THE last thirty years or so, reading was the most common form
of entertainment. These days, technology has been steadily replacing the
entertainment of reading a good book. According to a statistic from the
National Endowment for the Arts and the National Center for Educa-
tional Statistics, fewer than half (48 percent) of adult Americans read
literature for pleasure.

Reading on a regular basis, however, provides amazing benefits to the
health of our brain and our mental well-being. Compared to other
media—especially television—reading is an active process that engages
several parts of the brain, demanding much more from us neurologically.
As a result, reading makes you smarter and—even better—*keeps* you
smart as you get older, helping to protect against memory loss. It should
come as no surprise that the more you read, the more you increase your
vocabulary, general knowledge, spelling capabilities, and verbal fluency.[1]
Further, reading books or lengthy articles for an extended period of time
improves our focus, concentration, and attention skills.

Reading has the power to reduce stress, whereas other forms of media tend to increase stress. TV and the Internet require short bursts of attention and come with tons of distractions, noise, and fast-paced visuals. Reading for a protracted period of time, however, requires sustained attention with a contemplative attitude. Dr. David Lewis-Hodgson, of the Mindlab at University of Sussex in London, conducted a study that demonstrated how reading impacts our stress response. Subjects' stress levels and heart rates were increased through a variety of tests and exercises, and then they read for a mere six minutes. The results showed that reading reduced stress levels among participants by 68 percent, with some seeing stress levels lower than before they had started the experiment.[2]

Reading also enhances our creativity. As we read about new concepts, ideas, and information, we engage our imagination and are more creative in the real world. Although a book or story may provide lengthy descriptions of characters, plots, and scenery, our imagination and creativity bring them to life in our minds.

From a social standpoint, reading makes you a more informed and engaging person. No matter the genre you enjoy—novels, biographies, nonfiction, self-help, or any other—you always gain new knowledge and insight and something new to talk about with others.

✢ ✢ ✢

THE PATH TO CHANGE
READ AT LEAST TWENTY MINUTES PER DAY

READING IS A change you can enjoy anywhere at almost any time. Some tips:

SCHEDULE IT IN   Designate a block of at least twenty minutes during the day when you think you will have time to read. The longer the block, the more you will benefit. Reading at night before bedtime helps you wind down. Some enjoy reading during breakfast or lunch, others during their commute. Choose a time when you are least likely to be distracted.

GO FOR LENGTH   Although reading blog posts and short snippets in magazines may "feel" like reading, it isn't going to give you the amount of content that will allow you to fully reap the benefits of increased focus and concentration, relaxation, and stress reduction. Instead, opt to read books and articles of decent length.

CHOOSE FOR PLEASURE   Choose books and articles you *want* to read. Reading books or literature because you think you *should* will not be pleasurable. If you start a book and find your mind wandering or interest lacking for several days in a row, consider abandoning it for something you'll enjoy more. The more time you spend reading what you love, the more interested you will be in doing it.

EXPAND YOUR HORIZONS   Although you may be tempted to read romance novel after romance novel, broaden your horizons by exploring new genres. Not only will you learn more through exposure to new concepts, information, and vocabulary, but it may even help you develop new interests.

GO DIGITAL   With the influx of devices and eReaders, reading on the go has become easier than ever. You can instantly download a book, a magazine, or a newspaper any time you want. And if you are enjoying more than one book at a time, you can take your whole library with you.

HAVE BOOK, WILL READ   The easiest way to read more is to have something to read with you at all times. Bring a book, magazine, or eReader with you in your briefcase or purse. Keep a book in your car. Anytime you have five or ten minutes of downtime, such as at the doctor's office, you can squeeze in some reading.

CREATE A READING RITUAL   Create a ritual that makes you look forward to reading. Find a comfortable place with no distractions. You may enjoy reading on a park bench or at the beach or in the grass under a tree. Finally, consider sipping a beverage—such as green tea, a latte, or a glass of wine—or nibbling on a snack while you read.

SET A GOAL   Set a goal to read a certain number of books within a certain time frame. For instance, maybe you want to read two books per month or twenty-four books within a year. Whatever goal you choose, make sure it (1) is realistic and (2) doesn't take the fun out of reading. You want to remain inspired to read, not dread it as a chore. Go a step further and create a reading log to document each book you read, how long it takes, and your thoughts about it. Tracking your reading will give you a sense of accomplishment.

JOIN OR START A BOOK CLUB   Joining a book club offers many benefits. It provides you with a sense of community and the ability to make lasting friendships with people who share a common interest. Being part of a book club keeps you accountable to complete books, making you more likely to read on a regular basis. And being part of a book club gives you further intellectual stimulation because the books read are discussed and analyzed by the group.

READ TO CHILDREN   Reading to children benefits both parent and child. For parents, it provides an opportunity to spend focused quality time with your child. Children benefit from increased vocabulary, language, and speech development. Reading also prepares them for school and education advancement and develops listening and attention skills. It can also help them develop a passion for reading, as well as curiosity, creativity, and imagination. Discuss the books you read and ask them questions. If your children are older, create a family reading night. You could even create a "family book club" and choose the same book for all of you to read and discuss.

✢ ✢ ✢

GIVE ME A BREAK

The really idle man gets nowhere. The perpetually
busy man does not get much further.

—SIR WILLIAM HENEAGE OGILVIE

"IF I SKIP lunch and push through another hour, I'll get this work done."
Does this sound familiar? Although keeping your nose to the grindstone
may seem like a good way of staying productive, it can often backfire.
Research shows that skipping breaks can make us less productive and
reduce creativity, while increasing stress and exhaustion.[1]

Taking short, regular breaks allows your mind to refresh. Breaks give
your brain the rest it needs to feel reenergized and to refocus when
returning to a task. Essentially, a short break can act like a vacation
for your brain. When we spend too much time doing the same task or
working on the same problem, our minds can become "numb." We start
to lose focus and miss important details, contributing to slower speed,
decreased accuracy, and, if our job entails physical work, increased risk
of accidents. Giving the mind a break to think about nothing or something
other than work, however, gives it a chance to return with a new and
refreshed perspective.

Taking breaks improves productivity because it also gives the body and mind physical rest. Many of us sit and work at a computer or laptop for a good portion of the day. When we sit in the same position for too long, it can compromise our blood flow, which can negatively impact our oxygen and energy levels. Further, we become more susceptible to musculoskeletal pain and injuries, as well as eyestrain, fatigue, and tension in our back and neck, all of which contribute to decreased performance.

In short, building breaks into your workday should increase focus, concentration, and work speed, while decreasing stress.

✧ ✧ ✧

THE PATH TO CHANGE
TAKE REGULAR, SHORT BREAKS

TAKING BREAKS THROUGHOUT the day provides great benefits to your well-being. Here are some ways to make the most of your breaks.

DETERMINE YOUR NEEDS   Studies show that performance begins to deteriorate after fifty to sixty minutes of continuous work.[2] To avoid hitting this point, a break every forty minutes may be an ideal frequency to help eliminate a drop in productivity. Everyone is unique, however, so how often and how long your breaks should be depends on you as an individual. Experiment with different frequencies and lengths to find what works best for you. A word of caution: be sure not to take too many breaks, as that can be self-defeating and lead to procrastination!

DID YOU KNOW?

If you are especially short on time, consider a microbreak. In a 2003 study, it was found that a twenty- to thirty-second microbreak among data-entry workers increased their speed, accuracy, and performance.[3]

SCHEDULE BREAKS   In a 2001 study, researchers found scheduled breaks to be more effective than letting workers take breaks on their own.[4] Many of us get caught up in what we are doing and either forget to take a break or feel guilty for taking one. As a result, even when we need to get away from our work for a few minutes, we don't. Schedule in breaks so you can ensure you take them at optimal intervals.

TURN OFF WORK AND PROBLEMS   Although it might be tempting to think through a work problem during a break, try to shut off work-related thoughts. The goal of taking a break is to increase productivity by giving your mind a rest so you can return to work with a fresh perspective. Also, avoid thoughts that weigh you down or are negative, and instead focus on positive thoughts that are uplifting, invigorating, and inspiring.

MAKE BREAKS ACTIVE   In a 1997 study, it was found that short breaks that were active were more effective than rest breaks.[5] This is especially true if you hold a desk job. A little activity will increase heart rate, which in turn will increase oxygen flow to your brain and throughout your body. Some ideas:

Get some fresh air and a change of scene with a walk outside.

Stand up and take five minutes to stretch, either at your desk or in your office. Working from the top of your body down to your feet, stretch each muscle along the way.

When you need to use the bathroom, choose one on a different floor of your building and take the stairs.

Instead of emailing or calling a colleague in your building, walk to their office to speak with them.

Stand while speaking on the phone.

Walk to the cafeteria and get a drink or healthy snack.

If your office has a gym, exercise at lunch time.

OTHER THINGS TO DO   If getting up from your desk for five minutes is challenging, consider some of the following options you can do without getting up:

Meditate and breathe deeply Meditation and deep breathing can clear your mind, relieve stress, and help you refocus. First, turn off any distractions, such as reminders, your phone, or anything that could interrupt your meditation. Then, while seated at your desk, close your eyes and meditate while taking deep, cleansing breaths. Avoid thoughts of work and problems, and do your best to focus on your breath.

Read Opt to read something that has nothing to do with work to engage a different part of your brain. Keep a book at your desk. Pick up the newspaper. Flip through a travel magazine. Avoid reading on electronic devices, however, as they can strain your eyes and make your break less effective.

Listen to music Maximize relaxation by listening to songs that evoke a softer, more tranquil mood rather than the heavy or energetic.

Head to the water cooler A little socialization can go a long way to relieve stress. Chat about the latest play or theater production, a colleague's vacation, or even your favorite television show, for a little levity.

Take a nap More and more companies, such as Google, AOL, and Ben & Jerry's, encourage napping as a way for their employees to reenergize and refocus to increase productivity. If your office allows napping and you find napping restorative, take a ten- to fifteen-minute nap.

Enjoy a personal call Although personal calls are not something to overindulge in at work, making a personal call on your break might be just what you need. Call a friend or a family member to talk about something other than work topics or problems.

✦ ✦ ✦

FIRST QUARTER CHECKLIST

WEEKLY CHANGES	IN ACTION?
Week 1: Put Pen to Paper	☐
Week 2: Let the Music Play	☐
Week 3: Show Your Pearly Whites	☐
Week 4: Be a Goal Setter	☐
Week 5: Make Lists	☐
Week 6: Be a Mono-Tasker	☐
Week 7: Forget the Joneses	☐
Week 8: Meditate	☐
Week 9: Kick Indecision	☐
Week 10: Sip Green Tea	☐
Week 11: See the Best in Others	☐
Week 12: Read for Pleasure	☐
Week 13: Give Me a Break	☐

SILENCE YOUR INNER CRITIC

If you hear a voice within you saying, "You are not a painter," then by all means paint, boy, and that voice will be silenced.

—VINCENT VAN GOGH

ALTHOUGH A LITTLE constructive self-criticism can be beneficial—it motivates us to grow and become a better version of ourselves—too much of it, or the wrong kind, can be highly detrimental. We tend to be our own worst critics, and often we go too far. We forget our keys and think, "I'm such an idiot." Or we have an off day at work and think, "I'm incompetent." These negative thoughts become all too pervasive and can be highly destructive. They eat away at our ability to be happy, and they are at the very core of low self-esteem and self-confidence.

Self-talk is the constant stream of unspoken thoughts we think each day. Those thoughts can be either positive or negative, but negative self-talk is rarely constructive. Instead of providing helpful ideas for improvement, it focuses on what's wrong and is destructive. And when we allow ourselves too much negative self-talk for too long, it leads to stress and anxiety as well as depression. Positive self-talk, however, has the power to reduce stress and can lead to improved mood.

Negative self-talk tends to take on one of four forms: *catastrophizing*—you assume the worst is going to happen; *filtering*—you accentuate the negative and downplay the positive; *personalizing*—you assume you are to blame when things go awry; and *polarizing*—seeing everything as black or white, with no gray in between. You may put yourself down or call yourself names. Maybe you tell yourself you aren't good enough. Maybe you obsessively analyze personal interactions for evidence that people don't like you.

Often, patterns of negative self-talk start when we are children. Maybe a parent criticized you or led you to believe you were never good enough. Or maybe a parent suffered from lack of self-esteem, and you've come to model their behavior. Maybe you were made fun of in school. Or maybe you went through several damaging experiences that caused you to become sarcastic or negative. Regardless of the cause, these thought patterns will become more and more integrated into your way of thinking as you get older.

DUMP NEGATIVE THOUGHTS

Treating your negative thoughts as material objects may be an effective way to combat them. A study conducted in Spain found that when teens wrote down their negative body-image thoughts and then threw them away, their thoughts did not impact them later. When subjects were asked to keep their written thoughts physically in a safe place, however, they relied more on them later on.[1]

On the other hand, positive self-talk and positive thinking have been shown to provide tremendous benefit. Researchers believe they have the power to lower rates of depression and improve stress management.[2] These habits also help individuals improve their psychological and physical well-being and their coping skills during especially stressful times.[3]

✦ ✦ ✦

THE PATH TO CHANGE
MAKE SELF-TALK POSITIVE AND CONSTRUCTIVE

SHIFTING THE TONE of self-talk from negative to positive can vastly improve your well-being.

ACKNOWLEDGMENT   Negative self-talk can be so habitual, it can be difficult to recognize it or, for that matter, the damage it causes. The first step for this week's change is to become aware of any negative self-talk you do and to acknowledge that it hurts and is damaging. Use the Negative Self-Talk Assessment in Part III: Tools and Resources, and write down the negative thoughts that pass through your mind, along with the feelings they cause. Do your thoughts make you feel bad about yourself? Stressed? Sad? Angry? Also, document how these thoughts impact your life. Do they keep you from doing things you want to do? Do they impact your performance? Are your relationships affected— possibly making you vulnerable to abuse or disrespect from others? Any time a negative thought passes through your mind, journal your thoughts and feelings.

IDENTIFY THE REASON   Once you can identify when negative self-talk happens and how it makes you feel, try to understand *why* it happens. This requires some deeper introspection. Using the Negative Self-Talk Assessment, you can begin to understand where your patterns of negative self-talk developed. Knowing the cause can help you focus on the solution.

REFRAME NEGATIVE THOUGHTS   There are several things you can do to shift your thoughts from negative to more positive:

Stop sign When negative thoughts pop up in your mind, picture a big red stop sign and simply say "stop" to yourself. This visual and verbal cue will heighten your awareness of this behavior.

Speak to yourself as you would to others If you wouldn't say something to someone else, you shouldn't say it to yourself. Treat yourself with the same respect you accord others. Be kind, encouraging, respectful, and forgiving of your mistakes or faults, just as you might be to a child or loved one.

Ask how Negative self-talk can be highly limiting. It keeps us stuck and doesn't provide us with opportunities to grow and learn. If you are thinking, "I can't do this," or "I won't be successful," reframe the statement to be a question of "how," such as "How can I do this?" or "How can I be successful?"

Focus on the feeling Change a negative thought from a statement of supposed fact to one of feeling. For instance, if you had a bad week in which many things seemed to go wrong, stating, "I *feel* unlucky this week" is a slightly more positive way of saying "I *am* unlucky." Unlike facts, feelings are temporary, which allows us to have the thought without making it an absolute truth.

Focus on the moment Don't overdramatize a specific moment to represent your whole being or life. Instead, take that moment as what it is: just a moment. For instance, if you went on a blind date that went badly, think, "That blind date was not the best," instead of the more dramatic "I'm never going to find love."

LOVE YOURSELF UNCONDITIONALLY Loving yourself unconditionally is key to turning off negative voices in your head and accepting who you are, including your imperfections. All of us have our faults and are far from perfect. Holding yourself to extremely high standards—or worse, a standard of perfection—is unrealistic. Allow yourself to be wrong. Allow yourself to fail. Allow yourself to make mistakes. Be forgiving and kind.

KEEP AN ARSENAL OF POSITIVITY When negative thoughts creep in, sometimes a simple reminder of the positives can go a long way. Using your Negative Self-Talk Assessment, document five things for each of the following: (1) What you love about yourself, (2) your strengths, and (3) your accomplishments. Whenever the negative self-talk starts, refer to your journal to remind yourself of all of the positive things that make you the amazing person you are.

DO A REALITY CHECK   Just as what you might read in a tabloid is unbelievable, your self-talk, when put to the test, probably doesn't hold much water either. Any time you start to think negatively about yourself, ask: Am I *really* [fill in the blank]? When you stop to ask this question, you will likely see how overdramatic your thoughts are, and you will retract your statement. Conducting a simple reality check slows down your thought process so you can think a little more rationally and clearly and, ideally, more positively.

GIVE NEGATIVE THOUGHTS AN IDENTITY   It isn't nice to call names, but when it comes to your inner negative voice, doing so may lend some humor. When your inner voice obsesses over how everything is wrong, call it something like "Debbie Downer." Or if it harps on your mistakes and judges your competence, call it "Perfect Peter." Giving your inner voice a persona puts distance between you and your thoughts and allows you to categorize thoughts, making you aware of those that are repetitive and damaging.

✣ ✣ ✣

GO BEYOND YOUR COMFORT ZONE

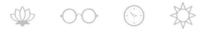

Opportunities to find deeper powers within ourselves
come when life seems most challenging.

—JOSEPH CAMPBELL

THE MORE WE live in our comfort zone and avoid challenges, the less likely we are to thrive. When we decide to take risks, however, we often find this leads to greater happiness, increased productivity and creativity, more success, and a greater sense of vitality.

When we do things that challenge us, something amazing happens: we feel more invigorated, excited, and alive than when we live with the status quo. When we push ourselves to do something that feels a tad uncomfortable or stretches us, we are forced to go past our limits and reach new and greater heights. As a result, we become capable of doing things we never thought we could. We become a better version of ourselves.

When we challenge ourselves, just as when we learn new things, we also develop new neural connections and encourage brain plasticity. And when there are positive outcomes, we gain a new perspective that challenges our traditional way of thinking. This helps keep us more youthful in both mind and spirit. We become more flexible and adaptable, making us better prepared for change and whatever unexpected challenges may come our way.

DID YOU KNOW?

The Grant Study at Harvard, conducted by Dr. George Vaillant, was a seventy-five-year longitudinal study of men from two different demographics: Harvard college sophomores from the classes of 1939 to 1944, and economically disadvantaged inner-city youths of Boston from 1940 to 1945. The study showed that for both groups, taking on challenges, despite setbacks, was one of the best predictors of long-term success in all aspects of life, including relationships, career, and health.[1]

Finally, taking on challenges helps strengthen self-confidence. The more you push yourself and are successful in what you take on, the more confident you'll feel about your abilities. With each risk taken, the boundaries of your comfort zone expand beyond where they were before you took the risk. Not only will you feel more inspired to take on future challenges, but they also won't seem so daunting.

✦ ✦ ✦

THE PATH TO CHANGE
TAKE ON CHALLENGES

ALTHOUGH IT MAY seem scary or uncomfortable, taking on challenges helps you be the best you can be and live the best life possible. Consider some of the following tips:

START WITH YOUR MINDSET   The ability to push out of our comfort zone relies on the belief that we can. In *Mindset: The New Psychology of Success*, psychologist Carol Dweck discusses how our mindset is what allows us to be successful or holds us back. With a *fixed* mindset, we believe our qualities or capabilities are fixed. When confronted with a challenge, we tend to give up easily. In a *growth* mindset, however, we believe we can continually grow and see challenges as opportunities to do so. We are open to failure and see it as part of the learning process, allowing us to try, try again until we succeed. Maintain a growth mindset by shifting thoughts of "I can't" to "I can."

LISTEN TO YOUR INNER VOICE   It is important to challenge yourself just enough so you feel a bit of trepidation, but not so much you overdo it. A very simple test is to listen to your inner voice as you respond to the challenge at hand. You should feel a little bit of fear along with some excitement. If, however, you feel calm and confident about the challenge, you may be setting yourself up for another version of your current situation. Or, if your response is fraught with anxiety or the idea makes you feel sick to your stomach, you may be pushing yourself a little too far.

START SMALL   You don't have to go through major risk taking right off the bat. If you aren't used to going out of your comfort zone, challenges such as launching your own business or jumping out of an airplane might be too much all at once. Instead, start small. Instead of skydiving, go parasailing. These challenges are a little less risky but make steps toward the bigger challenges.

UNDERSTAND YOUR COMFORT ZONE   According to Marcus Taylor, creator of the Comfort Zone calculator, there are three elements to your overall comfort zone, associated with different realms of activities: he calls them *adrenaline* (for example, skydiving), *professional* (for example, starting a new business), and *lifestyle* (for example, getting married). Each of us has a different level of comfort in each of these areas, and knowing where you have the least comfort might spark some ideas on where to challenge yourself. Using the Comfort Zone Assessment in Part III: Tools and Resources, assess where you could benefit from challenging yourself.

LOOK FOR OPPORTUNITIES EVERY DAY You don't necessarily need to go to an extreme to be challenged. Look at the different activities you do each day and think about how you might be able to change them so they push you a little further. For instance, if you have been running three miles, three days a week, for the last three years, challenge yourself by increasing your mileage or the number of days you run. Or, if you've been at the same job for several years and you are feeling bored, maybe it is time to speak to your boss about new opportunities within your company.

KEEP CHALLENGING COMPANY Seek out those individuals who value growth and enjoy being challenged themselves. They are more likely to be supportive and encouraging when you take on your own challenges. Naysayers and negative people, however, are likely to hold you back or keep you stagnant.

✢ ✢ ✢

GET MOVING

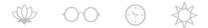

It is exercise alone that supports the spirits,
and keeps the mind in vigor.

—MARCUS TULLIUS CICERO

UP UNTIL THE twentieth century, most people lived very active lives.
They walked frequently, they used manpower instead of machine
power, and they relied on manual labor for their livelihoods. Today,
our level of activity has greatly diminished due to technology and
modern inventions. We have become an extremely sedentary species,
relying on treadmills and dumbbells to get a modicum of the activity
our ancestors once did.

No doubt we all know regular exercise is good for our physical health:
it facilitates healthy weight maintenance, assists in decreasing body
fat, and strengthens the heart and lungs by increasing heart rate and
oxygen intake. Staying active, however, also provides tremendous
benefit to our mental well-being. Studies show that regular activity
improves mood, reduces anxiety and depression, relieves stress, and
even improves memory.[1, 2]

The term "runner's high" refers to the release of endorphins—chemicals or neurotransmitters—in the brain during and shortly after exercise. Endorphins elevate mood, benefiting mental well-being, and increase happiness. If you prefer other types of exercise, you're in luck: endorphins are released as a result of *any* type of physical activity. And physical activity reduces levels of the stress hormones cortisol and adrenaline. This provides a natural distraction and break from the typical worries and stress of everyday life, helping you maintain a more calm and clear perspective. And although it may seem like a superficial perk, a fit and healthy appearance also has a direct and positive impact on our self-confidence, which in turn increases happiness, while lowering depression and anxiety.

Staying active also has a significant impact on the intellect. Aerobic activity increases oxygen to all the cells, including those in the brain and other organs. This increase in oxygen flow is vital to brain function, memory, and focus and concentration. In a 2007 study conducted by Scott Small of the National Academy of Sciences, a three-month program of intense aerobic exercise (one to two hours, four days a week, of intense aerobic exercise on a treadmill or stationary bike) produced a 30 percent increase in new neurons in the hippocampus, a part of the brain responsible for memory. Further, participants had improvements on tests of mental recall.[3] Other studies show that children who get as little as fifteen minutes of daily physical activity have improved concentration, memory, and classroom behavior, even more so than students who received an additional lesson.[4] This boost in cognitive function also holds true for adults. Older adults who walked for forty-five minutes at least three times per week were found to perform better in psychological tests than those who just did stretching.[5]

Exercise, when timed well, also improves sleep patterns. A 2010 study conducted by Kathryn Reid, Ph.D., of the Department of Neurobiology and Physiology at Northwestern University, showed sedentary adults who complained of poor sleep who were put on a regular exercise regimen for sixteen weeks went from being a "poor sleeper" to becoming a "good sleeper." They also reported decreased symptoms of depression and daytime sleepiness, as well as increased vitality.[6].

✢ ✢ ✢

THE PATH TO CHANGE
GET THIRTY MINUTES OF AEROBIC ACTIVITY, THREE DAYS PER WEEK*

IF EXERCISE IS new for you or you've struggled with it, you may not think of it as a fun, recreational release. The more you exercise, however, the more you will enjoy it. I promise.

GET THE FOUNDATION   If you are beginning from ground zero, the idea of exercising for thirty minutes, three times a week, may seem overwhelming and unappealing. To stay motivated and develop a liking for it, follow these ground rules:

Ease into intensity Do not launch into an extremely intense workout right from the start. This will likely lead to burnout and frustration. Instead, start with low to moderate intensity exercise that challenges you enough to elevate your heart rate but not so much that you struggle. Once you have been comfortably exercising for thirty minutes, three days a week, push yourself to increase the level of intensity so it is more challenging.

Step up the duration Start with three days and commit to a minimum of ten minutes of activity each day. The next week, add another five minutes to the duration until you reach thirty minutes per day. If carving a full thirty minutes out of your day is very difficult, consider breaking it up into two fifteen-minute blocks.

Simple is best Keep your exercise program manageable, practical, and simple. The more complicated you make it, the less likely you'll be to

*Always consult your doctor prior to beginning a new fitness regimen.

stick with it. If an activity requires too much planning, time, or coordination, you'll be less likely to do it, even if it is your favorite activity in the world. Reserve those activities that may require more effort (like skiing or snowboarding) for weekends, and make weekday exercise convenient and simple.

EXERCISE INTENSITY

Exercise intensity is an important factor of an exercise program. Ideally, you should reach 65 percent to 85 percent of your Maximum Heart Rate (MHR) for a minimum of twenty to thirty minutes.

The simplest method of evaluating exercise intensity without a lot of calculations is to conduct a talk test. If you can hold a conversation while exercising without any change in breathing, you are not exercising intensely enough. If, however, you're too out of breath to speak, you're probably overexerting yourself and should decrease your intensity. Push yourself enough so conversation is more difficult than usual, but not so much that it is impossible.

These basics will help you step up your pace and time so you feel comfortable and confident in taking on a longer, more difficult workout.

MAKE SEDENTARY ACTIVITIES ACTIVE One of the best ways to shift your mindset to one that is more active is to look for opportunities to turn sedentary activities into those that are more active. For instance, watch television while doing something that is more active, such as cleaning, doing laundry, or, yes, exercising. Sit on a medicine ball at work. Stand at your desk. Make business meetings walking meetings. Stand or walk around when talking on the telephone. Opt for the stairs instead of riding the elevator or escalator.

WALK IT OFF   Choosing to walk instead of driving or taking public transportation can make a big difference. Walking is one of the easiest and most beneficial ways to build activity into your life. Make walking a natural part of your commute or running errands. Look for small opportunities to squeeze in an extra few steps everywhere you go.

EMBRACE TECHNOLOGY   Track your activity each day. Most cardio machines provide details of your workout—time, calories, distance, and so on. If, however, you exercise outdoors or don't use machines, a standard pedometer can tell you how far you walk each day. Other devices allow you to keep track of other useful metrics, such as calories burned, the hours and quality of your sleep, the number of stairs you climb, and more.

DO WHAT YOU LOVE   One of the best ways to enjoy exercise is to do something you enjoy. If you don't like running, forcing yourself to run won't get you anywhere (pardon the pun). Go to a local college and see what physical education courses they offer, or explore your local parks and recreation department for outdoor activities in your area. Many local continuing education programs also offer exercise classes. So many activities can raise your heart rate; you'd be hard-pressed not to find *anything* you enjoy. Some ideas: walking, running, cycling, swimming, aerobic dance, rowing, hiking, in-line skating, pole-dancing, Zumba, belly dancing, karate, tae kwon do, boxing, racquetball, and tennis.

PLAN FOR IT   If making time for exercise each week is a challenge, schedule it into your calendar so you have no excuses. Block off time for the exercise itself, as well as any required travel, showering, and changing, so you don't feel time-constrained. Also, if you plan on exercising during the workday or after work, make sure to pack and take along any and all gear you'll need.

OPT FOR THE MORNING   For many of us, it is much easier to exercise in the morning, as we generally have no excuse for skipping it. If you wait until the end of the day, however, many excuses creep in: you are too tired, you have to work late, you have a client dinner, and so on.

MAKE IT SOCIAL   Exercise is much more fun when you enjoy it with a friend or a partner. Share a walk, a hike, a run, an aerobics class, or a bicycle ride with a friend. The only caveat in selecting a workout buddy is that you make sure you choose one who is as committed to exercise (if not more so) as you. Otherwise, you may find yourself continually motivating your friend or, worse, being talked out of exercising.

DIVERSIFY   Vary your activities to help minimize boredom or burnout. This will keep you engaged so you are more likely to stick with the program. Enjoying a variety of activities will also challenge your body and your mind in different ways too.

PARTICIPATE IN A RACE   A wonderful way to stay active, as well as motivated, is to sign up for races and events. You can go almost anywhere in the world to enjoy a race. If you like to run, consider a 5K, 10K, or marathon. If you enjoy cycling or swimming, look for races that involve those activities. And of course, if you are passionate about a cause or charitable organization, look for fund-raising athletic races in which you can participate. Some examples are the Avon or Susan G. Komen walks for breast cancer, or the American Diabetes Association's Tour de Cure.

✧ ✧ ✧

GIVE THANKS

The struggle ends when the gratitude begins.
—**NEALE DONALD WALSCH**

THE SIMPLE ACT of giving thanks means stopping to reflect on our life and express gratitude for all of the good things we have. When practiced on a daily basis, this act can have a tremendously positive impact on our overall mental well-being.

Regularly practicing gratitude means showing appreciation for our lives, our relationships, and our good fortune. Those who practice gratitude regularly tend to be happier than those who don't. They have a more positive, optimistic attitude and are more enthusiastic, joyful, and energetic. Additionally, they tend to be more generous, helpful, and giving in spirit.[1] Being thankful also helps reduce feelings of stress, anxiety, and depression. Gratitude acts as a buffer to the negative effects of stress, increasing resiliency and our ability to deal with everyday problems and recover from traumatic events more easily.[2]

Practicing gratitude can also positively impact our sleep patterns. Grateful people take less time to fall asleep, sleep more soundly and for longer durations, and feel more refreshed when they wake.[4]

DID YOU KNOW?

According to a study conducted by Robert Emmons, Ph.D.,
individuals who practice gratitude feel 25 percent happier
than those who don't and report greater optimism about
the future, better feelings about their lives, and about one
and a half hours more exercise per week.[3]

When we outwardly practice gratitude and express thanks to others, it
can help strengthen our relationships, making us feel more connected
and committed to other individuals—and in return making them feel
more connected to us. Being thankful helps promote forgiveness and can
increase feelings of satisfaction in relationships.[5]

Finally, practicing gratitude has been shown to be good for our overall
health. Studies show that gratitude can strengthen the immune system,
lower blood pressure, reduce symptoms of illness, aches, and pains, and
encourage exercise and better self-care.[6]

✦ ✦ ✦

THE PATH TO CHANGE
CULTIVATE A MINDSET OF GRATITUDE

GRATEFULNESS CAN BE cultivated easily with a few practices:

THE TOP FIVE LIST   Think about the five things you are most grateful
for and document your list so that it is accessible anywhere, at any time.
You may want to keep it on your smartphone, in your wallet, or in your
purse. When you are having a bad day or are thinking negatively, use the
list as a quick reminder of the things that are positive in your life.

KEEP A GRATITUDE JOURNAL   Just as it strengthens other aspects of
life, journaling is a very powerful tool in raising awareness of your

gratitude. Use the Gratitude Journal template in Part III: Tools and Resources and update your journal as often as possible with things for which you are grateful. Try to be detailed in your descriptions, savoring the little things. When you have days in which you feel less than grateful, read your journal to lift your spirits and remind you of all the good in your life.

VARY YOUR FOCUS   Although it is easy to acknowledge the same blessings over and over, such as our health and our family, doing so can undermine our ability to find new things for which to be grateful. To keep gratitude fresh and diversified: (1) each time you journal or express gratitude, find a new area of life on which to focus (for example, home, family, friends, health, or career); (2) use different methods to express thanks (for example, journal, write a letter, say a mantra, share with a friend, or write a blog post); and (3) get very specific about your thanks. For instance, although I'm broadly thankful for my health, today I could be thankful for my healthy heart; tomorrow I might express gratitude for my strong bones and muscles; and the next day, I could appreciate my young and creative mind.

SEE THE GOOD IN THE LITTLE THINGS   It is easy to be grateful for the bigger, more obvious things in life, but when we can appreciate the smaller things, we find a new and higher level of gratitude. Pay attention to your surroundings, environment, and everyday joys. Maybe you are grateful for a sunny, warm day. Maybe you are grateful for a snow day! Maybe you are grateful for a smile sent your way. Enjoy and revel in the small details of life.

EXPRESS TO LOVED ONES   Make an effort, at least once a week, to express appreciation to those you love. Although we don't necessarily mean to, it is human to take the people we appreciate the most for granted. Yet expressing thanks for the things they do, their support, and their love will make them feel good and make you feel even better. Make a concerted effort to thank loved ones openly and to verbalize how much they mean to you. By the same token, part of practicing gratitude is being able to accept appreciation and thanks from others. If someone expresses gratitude toward you, be receptive and appreciative. If you struggle to accept thanks for any reason, try to understand why.

PRACTICE GLOBAL GRATITUDE   Those of us who enjoy our freedom, a sense of peace and security, a job that helps us pay bills, and an ability to obtain the primary things we need to live—food, water, shelter, and clothing—are very fortunate. These "luxuries," however, can be easily overlooked or taken for granted. Take time to actively appreciate some of the everyday things that make life wonderful and all of the benefits that come along with it. Remember the many people in the world who are not so lucky, living with war, poverty, hunger, disease, and cruelty on a daily basis. Reflect on the good fortune you enjoy as a result of the hard work of those who have come before you, and of those who fight today to protect your rights and the life you live.

REFRAMING   Try to see the silver lining. For instance, instead of complaining about the rainy weather, see the rain as a positive part of growth and renewal for the plants and flowers that will spring up as a result. Or, if you have to work late, be thankful for your job and for the ability to make money and support yourself, or yourself and your family. Find ways to take the seemingly bad and see the good in it instead.

ENGAGE OTHERS   What goes around comes around. Asking others what they are thankful for can create good karma and good vibes among your family and friends. When your spouse or child comes home at the end of the day, ask what good things happened to them or what they are grateful for from their day. Or, when you see a friend for lunch or dinner, make a point of discussing your blessings of the week and having them do the same. Getting others to reveal what they are grateful for helps to spread joy and gratitude.

TEACH GRATITUDE TO CHILDREN   If you are a parent, godparent, aunt or uncle, grandparent, or teacher, try to instill the practice of gratitude in the children in your life. When children are taught to practice gratitude, good habits are instilled early for the longer term. Further, the benefits of practicing gratitude—increased happiness, joy, and optimism, and decreased stress, depression, and anxiety—are reaped at any age.

DEVELOP A RETROACTIVE PRACTICE   Developing a sense of gratitude from today forward is a great start, but acknowledging your past blessings can further boost your sense of gratitude and happiness. Think about those individuals who have helped you or had a particularly positive impact on your life and thank them. If you haven't spoken in some time, pick up the phone or write a letter and communicate your heartfelt thanks. Be as detailed and as specific as possible.

✦ ✦ ✦

PLACE VALUE ON DOING

> The person who has lived the most is not the one with the most years but the one with the richest experiences.
>
> —JEAN-JACQUES ROUSSEAU

ALTHOUGH MONEY SURE can make life easier, it doesn't necessarily equate to happiness. What you spend your money on, however, can make all the difference in the world.

Studies show that when individuals spend money on an experience, such as a meal with friends, a vacation, or even a day at the beach, they tend to feel happier than when they spend their money on a material possession, such as a car, a house, or a new gadget. What's more, the happiness derived from purchased experiences goes beyond the moment of the purchase itself. When an individual thinks about a past experience or anticipates one in the future, they feel more positive than when they think about a past or future material purchase.[1]

Spending our time and money on experiences rather than material possessions brings us greater joy for a variety of reasons. For starters, the joy our possessions provide is relatively finite and fades over time. Experiences, however, take longer to fully absorb, become greater in significance over time, and can provide us with a lifetime of memories. Further, possessions are what they are—they are concrete, whereas experiences are more abstract and often engage all of our senses. For instance, when we purchase a new car, we may feel happy for a week or a month, but eventually the car becomes commonplace in our lives and loses its specialness. When we go on a weekend getaway, however, we spend time with friends or family, taste new foods, see interesting sights, smell local scents, and become absorbed into a new environment—all of which give us endless opportunities to derive pleasure. And even when something negative occurs—such as getting lost in a strange city or dealing with bad weather on a trip—we tend to remember the best in those moments, focusing on how they made the experience that much more interesting or memorable.

DID YOU KNOW?

A 2010 Princeton University study found that emotional well-being closely correlates with an annual income up to about $75,000. Income beyond that level, however, doesn't translate into more happiness. On average, an American who earns $250,000 per year isn't likely to be any happier than one who earns $75,000 per year.[2]

Another reason spending on experiences is preferable to spending on material possessions is that experiences often have a social component: we are more likely to share our experiences with others, while our possessions are generally enjoyed by us and us alone.[3] When we experience things with other people, it increases our social connectedness, strengthens our relationships, and enables us to develop deeper and stronger bonds with others—all of which contribute to our happiness.[4]

❖ ❖ ❖

THE PATH TO CHANGE
CHOOSE EXPERIENCES
OVER POSSESSIONS

PLACING VALUE ON and investing in experiences provides us with a greater sense of vitality. Our experiences make us feel alive and give us greater opportunities to grow. Shift your spending habits to experiences by considering the following:

RAISE YOUR AWARENESS   Any time you consider purchasing a new possession, stop yourself and think about what kind of experience it will give you. Ask yourself: How much joy will this bring me? Will the joy be temporary or long-lasting? Will this purchase provide me with an experience that will be unforgettable? Will the purchase be something I can share with others? If it becomes clear the purchase will provide only short-term benefit to you, think about an experience you could purchase instead that would provide you with longer-term benefits. For instance, if you have your eye on a new pair of shoes for $150, ask yourself what kind of experience you could enjoy for that same amount. Maybe you'd enjoy a concert with friends or a dinner cruise during the summer. Once you think of an experience you'd enjoy, seriously consider diverting the money for the purchase from possession to experience.

SPEND ON EXPERIENCES YOU WANT   When choosing experiences, be mindful that spending on those you don't want is wasteful and may actually cause unhappiness. Further, just because your friends or family want to do something doesn't mean that you will too. For instance, if you tend to be low-key and casual, a really expensive dinner at a fancy restaurant may not be nearly as enjoyable as a dinner out at a local burger joint. Or, if you are adventurous, staying at an all-inclusive resort where you never leave the property might feel limiting as opposed to staying at an eco-resort that encourages off-property exploration. All experiences are not created equal, so be mindful of the experiences you value and those you don't, so you invest in those that will bring you the greatest joy.

BE INCLUSIVE   Because we get more out of our experiences when we share them with others, make a point of planning experiences with friends and family. Ask a friend to accompany you on a walk. Bring a family member with you to a show. Go with a colleague to a lecture.

PLAN IN ADVANCE   As mentioned earlier, the anticipation of our experiences can give us a great deal of pleasure as well. Plan experiences in advance so you can look forward to them and anticipate the happiness they'll bring.

MEMORIALIZE EXPERIENCES   Similarly, reminiscing about experiences keeps them alive in our minds and allows us to continue enjoying them even after they are over. Extend your joy with some of the following:

Take photographs Take photographs during the experience. Share them online afterward or gift friends who shared in the fun with photo albums so they can relive the experience for years to come too.

Journal Keep a journal or log to document what happens so you can read about it in detail in the future.

Create a summary video For bigger experiences, such as vacations or special occasions, use the photographs and videos you capture to create a summary video for friends and family.

CREATE AN EXPERIENCE FUND   If you have your eye on an excursion that could be very expensive, such as a trip to New Zealand or the Galapagos, create an "Experience Fund" in which you stash money away each week toward the cause. Do some research beforehand so you know how much you have to save and for how long. Be consistent in your efforts to save and, when appropriate, consider diverting funds you would have spent on material purchases to your fund.

KEEP AN EXPERIENCE BUCKET LIST   Although you may not have the money now to do each and every thing you'd like, one day you might. Start a bucket list of all the experiences you hope to have. When you think of something new, add it to your list.

LOOK FOR FREE ALTERNATIVES   Although certain experiences cost money (for example, vacations, concerts, meals), there are many experiences that are free. When you are given an opportunity to spend money, look for ways to enjoy the same or a similar experience by spending less money or, better yet, no money at all. For instance, instead of going out to dinner with friends, host a potluck dinner where everyone contributes by bringing a dish. Or, if you need a vacation, consider a "staycation" for a few days at home and explore your local surroundings instead of spending a lot of money on travel. And if you are looking for a music fix, see what free concerts or performances are happening in your local community instead of going to an expensive show.

THE GIFT THAT KEEPS ON GIVING   For birthdays and holidays, gift loved ones with experiences instead of possessions. Even if they were hoping for a specific item, such as a new gadget, they will likely appreciate the experience they have even more. You may even get them to shift their thinking to value experiences over possessions too. If you have an opportunity to gift or reward employees or coworkers for a job well done, give them a shared experience they can enjoy as a group. Shared experiences, especially, will help boost morale throughout your organization or team.

✤ ✤ ✤

SEEK SILENCE

Silence is a source of great strength.
—**LAO TZU**

FROM THE MINUTE the alarm goes off, signaling the start of our day, until our eyes shut at night for sleep, many of us are bombarded by noise—or in other words, unwanted sound. If you stop and listen, right now, you may notice people chatting, sirens blaring, traffic whizzing by outside your window, or, at the very least, the hum of a few appliances in the room. Noise is everywhere, and it is doing a number on our psyche.

When we are faced with too much noise, we experience a biological stress response. In one study, conducted during the closing of the old Munich Airport and the opening of the city's new airport, students in schools near both sites were evaluated before, during, and after the switch. Students in the school near the currently working airport had higher levels of the stress hormones adrenaline and cortisol, compared to students near the closed airport.[1]

Noise—which includes everything from horns honking on the street outside to loud conversations down the hall—disrupts our thought processes, impairs performance, and diminishes concentration. In the same airport study in Munich, students near the old airport initially scored lower on tests of memory and reading, but they improved once it was closed. The reverse occurred for the students at the new facility: their scores declined after the new airport was opened.[1] And when noise is truly excessive or reaches abnormally high decibels, it can lead to mental fatigue, anxiety, and even aggression.[2]

READING AND THE NOISY ENVIRONMENT

One study conducted in the 1970s showed that children living on lower, noisier floors of an apartment building in New York City had lower reading scores than those living on higher floors.[3] Noise's impact on reading was also observed in the school environment. Environmental psychologist Arline Bronzaft, Ph.D., conducted a study in New York City and found that reading scores of elementary school students whose classrooms faced train tracks were much lower than scores of those children in classrooms on the quieter side of the same school.[4]

Spending time in a quiet, calmer environment is therapeutic. It gives our brain the reprieve it needs and allows us to decompress. It gives us an opportunity to focus, without constant disruption, and delivers a bit of peace and quiet to our day (and night).

✦ ✦ ✦

THE PATH TO CHANGE
MINIMIZE NOISE IN YOUR ENVIRONMENT

WE HAVE GROWN so accustomed to living in a noisy world that it almost feels unnatural or strange when we are immersed in silence. When we can exist in a quieter environment, however, we feel more at ease, less stressed, and more focused. Make your environment more tranquil with some of the following tips:

ASSESS YOUR ENVIRONMENT   Using the Noise Inventory Worksheet in Part III: Tools and Resources, take inventory of your home and of your workspace at different times of the day to assess the noise level. Do you feel distracted? Do you feel stressed? Can you focus when working? Are there noises that can be turned off or diminished?

CREATE A QUIETER ENVIRONMENT   For especially loud spaces, look for ways to diminish the amount of audible noise. If, for instance, your appliances are old and tend to be loud, consider purchasing new ones with low noise ratings. Use soft fabrics to decorate, as softer textiles help with sound absorption. If you live on a busy street, consider replacing windows with those that provide noise reduction, or, at the very least, use window treatments that help reduce outside noise.

SPEND TIME IN NATURALLY QUIET PLACES   Instead of frequenting noisy places, choose quieter and more peaceful environments. When you need to concentrate on work, go to the stacks of a public library instead of a noisier and more distracting local coffee house. Instead of meeting a friend in a busy café, have a picnic in the park. Instead of going to a sporting event, enjoy time in a local park, at the beach, or at a nature preserve.

DID YOU KNOW?

Riding a snowmobile, listening to music with headphones at a high volume, playing in a band, and attending loud concerts can lead to noise-induced hearing loss. Approximately 15 percent of Americans between the ages of twenty and sixty-nine have hearing loss that may have been caused by exposure to loud sounds or noise at work or in leisure activities.[5]

TURN OFF THE NOISE   When noise is inevitable, you can physically turn it off with simple devices. For instance, if you work in a noisy workplace environment, the noise may increase your stress levels and diminish your ability to focus and remain productive. If you are lucky enough to have your own office, consider using a white noise machine to block out unwanted noise from outside. If you work in a cubicle, use noise-canceling earplugs. When you are traveling, use noise-canceling headphones or earplugs to shut out loud conversations or screaming babies, or even the overwhelming noise of the jet engines or the train rumbling on the tracks.

USE OF APPLIANCES   Minimize use of especially loud appliances—such as hair dryers, food processors, and vacuums—or consider using earplugs when you do. When watching television or listening to music, keep the volume low. You'd be surprised how low the volume can be and still be enjoyable.

QUIET NIGHT   Too many of us use television, music, video games, and other noisy distractions to fill the void of silence. So much so, that some of us even leave the television on for company or to fall asleep. Spending time in silence may sound scary, odd, or uncomfortable, but with practice it can provide wonderful benefits. One night a week, create a quiet night with minimal to no noise. If you live with others, have them take part in this ritual. Instead of watching television or listening to music, find quiet activities to enjoy, such as reading, playing cards, or sitting outside on your porch and listening to the crickets or the wind rustling through the trees.

✧ ✧ ✧

SPEAK UP

Courage is what it takes to stand up and speak;
courage is also what it takes to sit down and listen.

—WINSTON CHURCHILL

AS HUMANS, WE'VE been gifted with the ability to vocalize our thoughts and feelings, yet many of us choose not to put this gift to good use. There may be merit to keeping quiet in some situations, but, more often than not, speaking up can do us a greater service. Speaking your mind strengthens relationships, boosts self-confidence, releases stress, and even has the potential to accelerate your career.

The more we choose to remain silent, not voicing our emotions, feelings, ideas, or beliefs, the more we find it difficult to do so. It is an insidious cycle. Yet finding our voice and using it constructively can be incredibly rewarding. When you take the time to express yourself, you're not only authentically sharing with others so they can better understand you as an individual and where you are coming from, but you are also building closer connections. Further, studies show that by expressing yourself, you avoid pent-up anger, resentment, or stress, all of which can hurt relationships and even lead to disease, such as cancer, hypertension, and other major illness.[1]

Speaking up is important to building self-confidence and self-respect. When we keep things in, we inadvertently send a message that we have no opinion about the subject at hand. This can result in others' making decisions for us or dictating how we should think and feel. This can lead to a lack of trust in our own instincts and a loss of the ability to differentiate our own thoughts from what the rest of the world expects us to think. Speaking our mind takes guts, especially if what we have to say is unpopular. But the more you put yourself out there, the easier it will become, the more confident you'll feel, and the more self-respect you will gain.

DID YOU KNOW?

Several studies show that women are less inclined to speak their minds than men when in groups. One study out of Brigham Young University and Princeton University found that in a typical meeting women were likely to speak 25 percent less than male counterparts. This was especially true when women found themselves to be in the minority.[2]

Expressing yourself can also help you gain the respect of others. In the workplace, for instance, speaking at meetings and voicing ideas or solutions to problems shows you have something to add to the discussion and are capable of analytical thinking. If you choose to keep quiet, however, colleagues may not see your added value, and you may lose out on opportunities. On the other hand, if it is a personal matter about which you choose to remain silent, your silence doesn't give loved ones a chance to respond or to understand your viewpoint. And, worse, if what you want to say has the potential to positively impact the other person or your relationship, you are denying that opportunity to both of you. Verbalizing what's on your mind opens up pathways for change.

✣ ✣ ✣

THE PATH TO CHANGE
COMMUNICATE YOUR FEELINGS, THOUGHTS, AND IDEAS

IF YOU STRUGGLE to express yourself, this week's change may seem difficult. But it doesn't have to be. Consider the following to be most effective:

ASSESS YOUR WEAK POINTS   Identify when and in what situations you have the most difficulty expressing yourself. Is it at work? Is it with friends? Is it with family? Try to understand what about those situations or people causes you to keep quiet. Have past experiences molded you to remain silent? Do you fear the outcome of expression? Did speaking up in the past result in negative consequences? Use the Speak Up Assessment in Part III: Tools and Resources to address some of these questions and others that may help you better understand what holds you back from speaking your mind.

PRACTICE   If you are uncomfortable with speaking up, find low-risk ways to express yourself. If your soup is cold when it comes to the table at the restaurant, let the waiter know. If you prefer to watch a different movie than your partner does, tell him or her what movie you'd prefer to watch. The more you practice speaking your mind with smaller, inconsequential things, the more confidence you'll have to speak up and be assertive about more important things. Other ways to practice include joining a public speaking group, such as Toastmasters, a drama or other performance group, or a book club.

SPEAK UP, SPEAK RIGHT   Saying what needs to be said requires a delicate balance: do it too much and it can be just as detrimental as not doing it enough. If you are expressing feelings to a loved one or colleague, understand the intention behind what you have to say, especially if it might take the other person by surprise or be hurtful. Choose a time when both you and the other person will be open to the discussion.

Avoid speaking negatively of others or complaining. Speak with purpose and with constructive intent. Use "I" statements ("I feel" rather than "You make me feel") when explaining your position, so as to not put the other person on the defensive. Remain respectful and balanced, clear and concise. Finally, practice active listening so the other person can verbalize her thoughts, feelings, and opinions as well. This will make her feel involved, valued, and respected.

WHAT OTHERS THINK   Don't let the opinions of others stop you from asserting yourself. Sometimes what needs to be said will make others uncomfortable, annoyed, or downright upset. But saying what needs to be said, even if unpopular, may be exactly what is needed to change the course of your relationships, your career, your project, or whatever you're addressing, for the better.

FORGET PERFECT   If you don't speak your mind because you are worried that you won't express yourself perfectly or that the outcome won't be perfect, remember that speaking up is the first step to constructive dialogue. It is what will take you from point A to point B. If things are left unsaid, you run the risk of not being heard or understood at all. It is better to say something in a slightly awkward way to spark further discussion than to not have the discussion at all.

ENCOURAGE OTHERS TO SPEAK UP   As you grow more comfortable in sharing your feelings and viewpoints with others, encourage them to do the same. Getting others to speak their minds can help strengthen your relationships and help loved ones and colleagues communicate more effectively with you, so that you both gain a mutual understanding of one another, your feelings, and your viewpoints.

✧ ✧ ✧

PUT TIME IN A BOX

Make use of time, let not advantage slip.
—**WILLIAM SHAKESPEARE**

OVER THE LAST decade, the concept of "timeboxing" has become widely used in corporate America to increase productivity. It offers great benefits for personal time management as well. Timeboxing is a time management technique that limits the amount of time you spend on a task. Instead of working until completion, you work on something for a specific amount of time—say, thirty minutes—before moving on to something else.

The primary benefit of setting time limits to your tasks is that it boosts focus and productivity. According to Parkinson's law, the more time we are given to complete tasks, the more time it takes us to do them. When we are given a limit, however, we find ways to streamline processes and prioritize so we can finish the task on time. We are forced to focus and ignore distractions, making us much more productive. Further, productivity increases because we are forced to ignore time-wasting activities, such as checking email, surfing the Internet, or chatting on social media.

Time limits also help reduce procrastination and motivate us to take on distasteful tasks or projects. When we know we have to dedicate only a finite amount of time to something we don't enjoy (for example, taxes), it doesn't seem so terrible. This encourages us to take the first step toward completion. Even if we only make a dent in the undesirable project or task, we have at least made some progress, motivating us to continue toward completion.

Setting time limits also diminishes perfectionist tendencies. When we have all the time in the world to complete a task, it is easy to pore over every detail in the hope of making everything perfect. Before we know it, we've spent twice as long as needed. Time limits force us to finish, perfect or not.

When extremely large projects seem daunting or overwhelming, time limits help us break the task into more manageable subtasks. Not only is this a more productive approach, but we also feel like we are making progress toward the end goal with each smaller task we complete. Additionally, time limits encourage creativity by putting space between smaller tasks so we can reflect on the work done and return to the project with fresh perspective.

Finally, creating time limits for your work also gives you an opportunity to see how much time it takes you to complete certain tasks and projects. This increased awareness is helpful with scheduling and planning, better preparing you to say yes to projects you know you can accomplish and no to those that are unimportant or unrealistic.

✤ ✤ ✤

THE PATH TO CHANGE
SET TIME LIMITS TO YOUR WORK

SETTING TIME LIMITS can be useful for almost any type of work or task you want to accomplish. Everything from doing household chores to putting together a presentation at work can benefit. Here are some helpful tips to make time limits most effective:

USE A TIMER   As silly as it may sound, invest in a timer that can keep you on schedule. You can use anything you want: an old-fashioned alarm clock, a kitchen timer, your phone, or your computer. Whenever you begin a task with a time limit, set the timer and work until the alarm rings. Avoid the temptation to check the time while you are working; instead, trust that the timer will let you know when your time is up.

CHOOSE TASKS   You can put a time limit on any type of activity; however, you might find that it is most useful for the following types: those that require extra motivation because they are unpleasant or distasteful, such as doing your taxes; those that are very large or daunting, such as a big project at work; and those that can creep into "overtime" very easily, such as social media, reading or watching the news, and personal email.

SET APPROPRIATE TIME LIMITS   Set time limits that are appropriate to the task, as well as optimal for maximizing your personal productivity. For instance, if a task is boring or unappealing, such as paying bills, a shorter time limit of fifteen to twenty minutes might make the task seem less painful and motivate you to get started. On the other hand, if a task is part of a larger project and requires deeper focus and concentration, you might want to set a longer time limit of forty-five minutes to an hour so you can make real progress. The important thing is that the time limit be fitting; not so short that nothing gets accomplished, but not so long that you become burned out by a difficult or tedious task.

EXCEPTIONS   Although adhering to your time limits is important, there may be days when you are nearing the end of a time limit and feel inspired to keep going. This is called a "zone of productivity" or "flow." If you're on a task that is distasteful, requires creativity, or is part of a larger, more complicated project, embracing these times and continuing your work may be beneficial. Extend your time limit for a specific period (for example, a half hour) so you can accomplish more, but reevaluate your productivity level at the end so as to not waste any time if your productivity starts to wane. Taking advantage of these highly productive moments helps to offset those times when you are less inspired or fruitful. And, of course, if you do extend your time limit on a task, be sure to make adjustments to other tasks.

TIME LIMIT WITH OTHERS   Meetings and phone calls can quickly become ineffective and unproductive when they go on too long or are hijacked by someone who has no concept of time. Although you never want other people to feel disrespected or devalued, putting strict time limits to your meetings and phone calls can be helpful. The more consistent you are with your time limits, the more others will come to respect them.

✦ ✦ ✦

EAT GOOD FATS

Let food be thy medicine and medicine be thy food.
—HIPPOCRATES

WHEN IT COMES to our health, there is no denying that good nutrition is important to a fit, healthy body. But what you eat also has a huge impact on your brain.

The human brain is approximately 60 percent fat, so consuming the right fats is important to brain function. Diets high in trans fats and saturated fats from animal sources have been linked to a higher risk of dementia, depression, and cognitive deficits, while those rich in unsaturated fats are associated with both a lower risk for mental health issues and improved cognitive function.

Fatty fish, such as wild salmon, sardines, and herring, provide brain-boosting omega-3 essential fatty acids. Through their role in the production and maintenance of brain cells, omega-3s are especially helpful in lowering risk of dementia, depression, and cognitive decline, and improving focus and memory.[1, 2] Because essential fatty acids are not produced in the body, we must get them through our diet. Fish is the best source, as it contains both EPA and DHA forms, both of which are less available in plant sources. Shrimp and other shellfish also tend to be rich in vitamin B12, which is important to healthy nerves and brain cells and is linked to preventing depression.[3]

DID YOU KNOW?

When studies compare mental health disorders across countries, those populations with the highest fish consumption have the lowest rates of depression, bipolar disorder, and seasonal affective disorder, among other mental health issues.[4]

Nuts and seeds, which tend to be rich in vitamin E and contain free-radical–fighting antioxidants, have been shown to boost cognitive function. Due to their high content of plant-based omega-3 fatty acids, walnuts have been praised as one of the best varieties to enjoy. In a 2011 study, college students who consumed two ounces of walnuts in banana bread for eight weeks showed an improvement in inferential reasoning, compared to students who ate plain banana bread.[5] Other research, published by the *Society for Neuroscience*, found diets made up of 2 percent, 6 percent (a typical serving size of approximately one ounce or a quarter cup), or 9 percent (one and a half ounces) walnuts, were found to reverse brain aging as well as motor and cognitive deficits.[6]

Avocados and olives (and their respective oils) are rich in monounsaturated fats. Monounsaturated fats help maintain the structure of the brain cell membranes, and they promote healthy blood flow, which increases oxygen to the brain and lowers blood pressure, both of which are important to cognitive function. Research shows avocado and olive oil consumption can improve memory and ward off cognitive decline.[7] In a 2012 study of 6,200 healthy women over the age of sixty-five, the women who had the highest monounsaturated fat intakes had the best cognition test scores, on average, compared to those who consumed mostly the polyunsaturated fats found in corn and vegetable oils. Further, those women who had diets high in saturated fats had brains that appeared five or six years older than their biological age, whereas those who consumed the highest monounsaturated fat had brains that appeared six or seven years younger.[6] An added benefit of avocados and olive oil is that they're also both rich in vitamin E.

Finally, eggs provide a high-quality protein rich in amino acids, which are essential to the production of neurotransmitters. They are also rich in vitamin E and choline, a nutrient in the vitamin B family. Choline aids in the construction of acetylcholine, a neurotransmitter that is critical to memory and has been shown to improve long-term memory and attention-holding capacity, while reducing signs of dementia.[8, 9]

✤ ✤ ✤

THE PATH TO CHANGE
ENJOY BRAIN-BOOSTING FATS AND PROTEINS

THE FOODS MENTIONED in this week's change are quite versatile and can be easily incorporated into most diets.

A LITTLE GOES A LONG WAY   When consuming foods rich in healthy fat, such as nuts, seeds, avocados, and olive oil, remember that they are also rich in calories, so consuming them in moderation is key. Typical serving sizes are about an ounce of nuts or seeds (no more than a quarter of a cup), a quarter or half avocado, or a tablespoon of olive or avocado oil. When preparing a meal, avoid the temptation to enjoy all of these in one sitting, as the fat content can add up very quickly.

SIMPLY SALMON   Always opt for wild Alaskan or sockeye salmon. Not only will you be getting a bigger boost in omega-3s than from other fish, but you'll also be avoiding exposure to the potentially high levels of mercury found in swordfish, tuna, and other larger fish varieties. Choosing wild Alaskan or sockeye salmon will also help you avoid PCBs (polychlorinated biphenyls), typically found in other varieties of salmon, including farm-raised varieties. Opt for poached, grilled, or baked salmon, and avoid fried at all costs. If you don't like fish or salmon, consider taking omega-3 supplements rich in EPA and DHA.

NEW TAKES ON TUNA

Love tuna salad? A tasty and healthier option for cold tuna salad is to replace the tuna with water-packed canned Alaskan pink or sockeye salmon. Mix with a quarter cup of fresh avocado, Dijon mustard, lemon juice, and minced onion. Absolutely delicious!

If you prefer the hot version, create an extra brain-boosting salmon burger by mixing canned salmon with raw egg and whole-wheat bread crumbs, then baking.

SHRIMP AND SEAFOOD   Shrimp and seafood mix very well with pastas and rice. Try an Italian cioppino or Spanish paella, which often contain shrimp and other vitamin B12–rich seafood, such as mussels, oysters, and scallops. Add shrimp to a salad, or enjoy a bowl of freshly steamed mussels or clams. Avoid fried seafood, as it contains unhealthy trans fats.

GO NUTS, BE SEEDY   Walnuts and seeds can be enjoyed in countless ways. A few ideas:

Snacks Pair a handful of walnuts or seeds with a piece of fruit for a well-balanced snack that is high in fiber and vitamins and minerals.

Salads Sprinkle a tablespoon or two of chopped walnuts or choline-rich sunflower seeds on top of your salad.

Breakfast Top cereal, oatmeal, and nonfat Greek yogurt with a tablespoon of chopped walnuts or omega-3–rich ground flaxseed.

Sandwiches If you like PB&J sandwiches, replace the peanut butter with walnut butter. If you are adventurous, try making your own!

Side dishes Add walnuts and seeds to vegetables, stuffing, and casseroles.

Dessert and baked goods If indulging in dessert or enjoying bread, choose those made with walnuts, poppy seeds, or sesame seeds.

OLIVES, AVOCADOS, AND THEIR OILS Olives are especially versatile in pasta dishes, casseroles, and Mediterranean food. For salads, make your own dressing when possible and use either avocado or extra-virgin olive oil (EVOO). EVOO is the purest and most healthful variety of olive oil. Add a quarter or half avocado to smoothies to make them creamy, to sandwiches instead of mayo, and to salads as a topping. When cooking, use avocado oil for higher-heat dishes, such as stir-fries, and use olive oil in lower-heat cooking, such as low-heat sautéing.

EGGS Enjoy a scrambled egg or two for breakfast or a hard-boiled egg at lunch. Although eggs used to get a bad rap for their high cholesterol content, new research shows that eating eggs as part of a healthy diet does not lead to high blood cholesterol.[10] However, animal-sourced saturated fat and trans fats do. If you don't have high cholesterol, consuming eggs shouldn't be a problem.

MAKE A NIGHT OF IT Enjoy a variety of brain-boosting nutrients by having appetizers or tapas, each with a unique ingredient. Some ideas: salmon maki rolls rolled in sesame seeds, BBQ shrimp skewers, guacamole, deviled eggs, olive tapenade, and spiced walnuts. Teach friends and family how to make meals brain healthy by hosting a potluck dinner: Give each guest a unique ingredient to incorporate. You may end up with some new and tasty recipes.

✦ ✦ ✦

OPEN YOUR MIND

The quality of your life is in direct proportion to the
amount of uncertainty you can comfortably deal with.
—TONY ROBBINS

MANY OF US have grown up with certain values and beliefs that stay with
us throughout our lifetimes. These values and beliefs make us who we
are, and for the most part they are the foundation from which we make
decisions and live our lives. As important as it is to stay true to our
values, if our belief system is too rigid it can hold us back. When our
beliefs keep us from being open to new experiences, new ideas, or new
ways of doing things, we miss out on so much that life has to offer. So it
pays to cultivate an open mind.

When we are open-minded, we build stronger, closer relationships. Openness makes us better listeners and more empathetic, and even when we
disagree with someone, we can see their perspective and point of view.
When we are open-minded, we are more capable of patience and are less
disturbed by those who are different from us. And we are less judgmental
and more understanding of people's individual situations and needs. As a
result, people are more comfortable communicating with us, they trust
us more, and they feel respected, all of which makes us more attractive.

Having an open mind is important to managing stress. We are less inclined to get aggravated, frustrated, or upset when things don't go as planned and are more open to uncertainty. We are more flexible and can embrace outcomes that may not be what we expected; and we can accept that everything happens for a reason, which allows us to let go of the things we can't control. And when problems do arise, open-mindedness encourages more effective problem solving. We are open to hearing new and different ideas, and we can see solutions and possibilities we might not otherwise see.

Being open-minded also makes you a happier, more positive person. With an open mind, you are more inclined to see the good in a bad situation. Your openness allows you to experience new things, which might bring about interesting and exciting opportunities. When open-minded, you can more easily accept criticism and see negative experiences as chances for growth, allowing you to change aspects of your life or yourself that inevitably will lead you to greater happiness and fulfillment.

When you have an open mind, the world will open itself up to you. You'll be able to see the bigger picture more easily; you will have more fun and be more creative, and you can take pleasure in the unexpected.

✣ ✣ ✣

THE PATH TO CHANGE
ADOPT AN OPEN-MINDED ATTITUDE

ALTHOUGH YOU MAY have lived most of your life with a belief system and a set of values that have remained rather constant, you can still cultivate an open mind. Here's how:

VALUES VERSUS OPEN-MINDEDNESS   Don't feel you are abandoning your values or are changing who you are by having an open mind. Remember, you should always stay true to yourself. That said, being open to others' different ways of being, to new experiences, and to new ways of thinking broadens your mindset and provides you with richer and more amazing opportunities.

TAKE INVENTORY   None of us want to think of ourselves as judgmental, opinionated, or prejudiced. Yet many of us can have these characteristics in our makeup at one time or another. Take a step back and think about how you are as an individual and the origin of your thoughts. What perspectives might benefit from change? Answer the questions in the Open-Mindedness Assessment in Part III: Tools and Resources, to raise your awareness about areas on which you might consider focusing.

GET THE FACTS   When you are confronted with a situation in which you can feel yourself jumping to a conclusion, take a step back and question your thoughts. Ask yourself if you know for certain that your opinion or conclusion is absolutely correct. Is there another possibility? Is there another solution? Is there another explanation? Get all the facts about a person or a situation before forming an opinion.

LISTEN   To keep an open mind, you have to practice good listening skills. When we can listen with intention and really hear what others have to say, we can learn a great deal. The more we speak, however, the less we can remain open to other viewpoints. Practice active listening at least 70 percent of the time.

EMBRACE UNCERTAINTY   When you can embrace and accept uncertainty in your life, you free yourself from the burden of expecting everything to work out perfectly. As we all know, perfection doesn't exist. Understanding that there are many possible outcomes to a situation, and that all of them can work, is paramount to happiness. Believe in your ability to cope and adapt to changing circumstances, and move forward with confidence.

SEEK OTHER PERSPECTIVES   To cultivate an open mind, you need to expose yourself to new opinions and ideas. Talk to friends, family members, and colleagues about a variety of topics. Start with those that are relatively innocuous. For instance, talk about a new movie or a new restaurant. Get comfortable listening to people's thoughts and opinions on various subjects, and then take it to the next level. Engage in discussions with people on more emotionally driven topics, such as politics or religion. Practice your active listening skills and fight the urge to feel defensive or argumentative. Instead, listen with an open heart.

EXPOSE YOURSELF Open-mindedness is easier to cultivate when you gain exposure to different cultures, religions, and regions of your own country, as well as other countries. Go outside of your comfort zone and explore. Meet new people from different backgrounds and engage in deep conversations. If you are able to, travel to a new country every year or two, immerse yourself in the local culture, and avoid typical tourist hotels, restaurants, and tours. If travel is difficult, take continuing education classes about other cultures.

✢ ✢ ✢

SLEEP

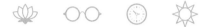

It is a common experience that a problem difficult at night is resolved in the morning after the committee of sleep has worked on it.

—JOHN STEINBECK

IF YOU ARE a parent, you most certainly understand the importance of sleep. It becomes vitally clear when your child doesn't sleep enough: he becomes fussy, cranky, and difficult to manage. There's good reason for this: sleep is extremely vital to our mental well-being—both in the short term and, even more so, in the long term. Sleep is so important to our brain development and function that the sleep quality we get, even as an infant, can determine much about our mental well-being as children and adolescents and even into adulthood.

Healthy sleep includes two distinct states—non-rapid eye movement (NREM) and rapid eye movement (REM)—that alternate in cycles and reflect differing levels of brain activity. They cycle over and over again during the night, with each complete sleep cycle taking about one and a half to two hours.

Getting adequate sleep is vital to proper cognitive function. When we don't get enough, we experience low energy levels and an inability to focus and concentrate. While we're asleep, the brain is busy processing the day and making connections between memories, events, what we've learned, sensory input, and feelings. REM sleep, especially, plays a significant role in these areas. REM helps with "memory consolidation," which involves the brain's committing new information to memory. When sleep is disrupted or we don't get enough, this process is interrupted and our ability to learn and remember things can diminish.

DID YOU KNOW?

A 1983 sleep study conducted in Canada showed children with a superior IQ had greater total sleep time—thirty to forty minutes longer each night—than children of average IQ and similar ages.[1]

Sleep also has a tremendous impact on our mood, stress levels, and happiness due to its role in maintaining proper hormone balance. If we skimp on sleep, our levels of serotonin (happy hormone) and melatonin (a hormone regulating the sleep-wake cycle) can drop, and cortisol (stress hormone) can increase, which can result in irritability, impatience, depression, moodiness, and other mental health issues.

When we suffer chronic sleep deprivation, the long-term impacts are undeniable. Medical complications may include high blood pressure, heart attack, heart failure, stroke, psychiatric problems including depression and other mood disorders, attention deficit disorder (ADD), and mental impairment. If you are sleep-deprived while pregnant, fetal and childhood growth retardation may result.[2, 3]

In summary, a good night's sleep can do wonders for you mentally.

✤ ✤ ✤

THE PATH TO CHANGE
GET SEVEN TO EIGHT HOURS OF QUALITY SLEEP PER NIGHT

STUDIES SHOW THAT sleeping seven to eight hours per night is optimal for your physical and mental well-being.[4] Here are some tips to ensure you get your prescribed shut-eye:

CREATE A SLEEP SANCTUARY   Make your bedroom a "sleep zone" conducive to healthy sleep habits. Some things to consider:

Mattress and pillows Your mattress and pillows are extremely important to a good night's sleep. If they don't support you comfortably, you may have trouble falling asleep or wake up feeling sore or unrested. Test different mattresses and pillows to find what works best for you. If the ones you like are expensive, seriously consider spending the extra money, as it is an important investment in your mental (and physical) health.

Sheets, linens, and pj's Similar to your mattress and pillows, your linens should be comfortable as well. Before purchasing, feel the fabric to make sure it feels the way you want. Often, higher thread counts are softer against the skin and more comfortable than lower thread counts, but be wary of a very high thread count at a low price; other factors are important too. When it comes to comforters, choose one most appropriate for your climate. Similarly, choose sleepwear that is appropriate for your climate, comfortable, and nonrestrictive.

Temperature and humidity Keeping your room too cold or too hot, too humid or too dry can disrupt sleep patterns. Moreover, we are less able to regulate our body temperatures when we sleep. Studies show that keeping bedroom temperatures on the cooler side—optimally between 60 and 68 degrees Fahrenheit (assuming sheets, sleepwear, and a comforter are used)—is best.[5] If you live in a dry climate, use a humidifier to make the moisture level of the room more comfortable. Likewise, if your room is uncomfortably humid, use a dehumidifier to remove some of the moisture from the room.

Pure sleeping zone Technology tends to excite us, preventing us from winding down when it is time to sleep. Make your bedroom a pure sleeping zone, meaning it shouldn't be used for work or for entertainment. Resist the urge to have a television or computer in your bedroom. Further, keep work materials or papers and wireless mobile devices outside of the bedroom, especially when it is time to sleep.

Lighting Put dimmer switches in your bedroom or use three-way bulbs that allow you to modify the light at night. Dimming light signals our brain that we are nearing bedtime. Also, make sure there are no distracting lights that might disrupt your sleep patterns. For instance, if you use an alarm clock, set the clock's brightness to the lowest level possible and move it away from your bed and out of view. Use blackout curtains to block out any and all light from the outdoors. If you still find minimal light disruptive, an eye mask may be helpful.

Noise Outside noise, even rain hitting the window, can be enough to disrupt sleep and keep a light sleeper awake. If you struggle with noise, consider sleeping with earplugs or buying a white noise machine to mask unwanted noise.

GET INTO A SLEEP SCHEDULE   Good-quality sleep relies on repetitive habit. Go to sleep at the same time each night and wake up at the same time each morning, even during weekends. Staying up too late and/or sleeping in can have a negative effect on your ability to maintain a quality sleep schedule and may even lead to insomnia. Maintaining a repetitive schedule, however, will keep your circadian rhythms (rhythms present in sleeping and feeding patterns of humans) in order. If you are currently struggling to get a minimum of seven to eight hours of shut-eye each night, start adding in sleep by going to bed fifteen minutes earlier or getting up fifteen minutes later than you do now. Do this every few days until you have reached seven to eight hours of sleep per night.

LET THE LIGHT GUIDE YOU   Ideally, you want to wake up with sunshine and go to bed when it is dark. This supports your circadian rhythms. Depending on where you live and the time of year, however, it may not always be possible. To compensate for these changes in day length, expose yourself to bright light in the morning when you wake and minimize exposure in the evening to signal your brain that it is time to sleep. You may even consider purchasing a "sunshine simulator" as your alarm clock. This type of alarm clock simulates sunrise by gradually increasing light in your room as you near your wake-up time.

EXERCISE   Studies show that regular exercise can improve sleep quality.[6] That said, it is important to time exercise well. Exercising too close to bedtime can keep you awake. A good rule of thumb is to exercise no closer than five to six hours before going to bed to avoid disrupting sleep patterns.

THINGS TO AVOID BEFORE BEDTIME   Be aware that the following stimulants and substances can sabotage your efforts to fall asleep.

Caffeine after 2 p.m.   Although they affect each individual differently, caffeinated beverages act as a stimulant and can keep you awake. The worst culprits, of course, are caffeinated beverages such as coffee, tea, and soft drinks. However, chocolate, diet drugs, over-the-counter allergy and cold medications, and some pain relievers can have caffeine in them as well.

Late afternoon naps   Naps can disrupt sleep patterns if taken too late in the day or for too long. Aim to keep naps no longer than forty-five minutes and try to take them before 3 p.m.

Medications   Many medications are known for disrupting sleep patterns. If you are on any medications and are experiencing difficulties getting good-quality sleep, speak with your doctor to see if any of the medications you are taking might be to blame.

Alcohol Although alcohol can most definitely make you sleepy, it inhibits your ability to get quality sleep throughout the night. Alcohol can hinder deeper stages of sleep and the crucial REM stage so important to your mental well-being.

Smoking Beyond the fact that smoking is unhealthy to begin with, smoking also causes sleep disruption. Many smokers sleep very lightly and often wake up in the middle of the night or early in the morning due to nicotine withdrawal.

Large meals, processed sugar, and beverages within two hours of bedtime
Consuming large meals or foods to which you are sensitive before bedtime can cause heartburn, indigestion, and discomfort, all making it difficult to fall asleep. Eating sugar or sweet foods close to bedtime raises your blood sugar, which also makes it difficult to fall asleep. Further, if you do happen to fall asleep, you may wake up and have problems going back to sleep when your blood sugar levels drop. Similarly, drinking a lot of fluids before bedtime will likely mean getting up in the middle of the night to empty your bladder at least once, if not several times.

Computer, television, video games, and other technologies All of these can fire up your brain prior to bedtime. Avoid television and other stimulating technologies for at least an hour before sleep.

Work If you tend to bring work home at night, stop working an hour to two hours prior to bedtime. This will give your mind a chance to relax and let go of the stresses of deadlines and other work-related issues.

THINGS TO ENJOY BEFORE BEDTIME Just as some things may keep you awake, there are things you can do to help promote sleep. Create a relaxing bedtime ritual that signals your mind and body it is time to wind down.

Drink a small cup of herbal tea about an hour before bedtime.

Enjoy a warm bath, hot shower, steam, or sauna—the heat will melt away stress and relax your muscles, preparing you for rest.

Listen to relaxing music or sounds of nature.

Meditate or breathe deeply.

Read a book (preferably one that isn't stimulating, such as a thriller or mystery).

Use aromatherapy—lavender is especially relaxing and soothing.

Enjoy a massage—if you don't have a partner who can indulge you, consider purchasing a massage chair or recliner that allows you to enjoy massage on your own. You can also look for small, inexpensive tools, such as "The Tingle" to massage your scalp, wooden foot rollers for your feet, or circular wooden massagers for your shoulders and other stress points on the body.

Journal—When we can't fall asleep, it is often because our mind is racing with all of the "have-tos" and events of the day. Journaling helps get the thoughts out of our head so we can relax.

WHEN SLEEP IS HARD TO COME BY   If there is a night when you can't fall asleep, or you wake up in the middle of the night and you find it difficult to fall back to sleep, don't lie in bed. Get up and do something that relaxes you or takes your mind off whatever is keeping you awake. Stay in dim light, but do something relaxing, such as reading, writing in your journal, or listening to relaxing music.

WHEN TO SEEK HELP   If you have trouble falling asleep on a regular basis, find yourself waking up each night, or feel fatigued or tired after a solid night's sleep, you may suffer from a sleep disorder. Sleep apnea, heavy snoring, and breathing issues during sleep can disrupt your sleep and create various problems. If you feel you are suffering from chronic sleep deprivation, seek out the help of a sleep specialist or speak to your primary care physician.

✤ ✤ ✤

GIVE YOURSELF A TIME-OUT

No man can think clearly when his fists are clenched.
—GEORGE JEAN NATHAN

PUTTING YOUR CHILD in a time-out as a form of discipline involves a temporary separation from an environment and/or other people as a way to help a child understand that her behavior has been inappropriate or unacceptable. Whether or not you agree with time-outs as a parenting style, using them for yourself may be a healthy way to get separation from challenging or difficult situations so you can gain perspective and remain in a positive, rational, healthy frame of mind.

When we are confronted with situations that negatively affect our mood, whether they cause anger, resentment, fear, pain, or sadness, it is easy to let our emotions get the best of us. When we are highly emotional, we can lose sight of the bigger picture and may struggle to engage in constructive or helpful interactions. We may say or do things that are hurtful or that we may come to regret. This can damage our relationships or create bigger problems than we originally faced. Giving ourselves time and separation from the situation, however, enables us to regain our composure so we can reengage in a more productive and rational way.

When we are emotionally charged, we often use anger to mask what we are really feeling. We use anger to hide our more primary and deeper emotions, such as sadness and fear, which doesn't allow for true resolution to occur. Separating yourself from an emotionally upsetting situation gives you the space you need to better understand what you are truly feeling so you can more clearly articulate your emotions in a logical and less emotional way.

A time-out also helps spare innocent bystanders. When confronted with situations that don't allow us to deal with our emotions or that cause us to suppress them, we may transfer those feelings to other people or situations at a later point. For instance, if you had a bad day at work because you lost a big client, you may suppress your feelings at the office, only to find that you release them by getting into a fight with your kids or spouse when you get home later that evening. Clearly, your anger didn't originate at home, but you released it there. When you take the appropriate time to digest and analyze your feelings, you can mitigate hurting or upsetting other people who have nothing to do with the situation.

Take a time-out when needed so you can avoid emotionally charged behavior that may have longer-term negative impacts on your relationships, stress levels, and overall happiness.

✢ ✢ ✢

THE PATH TO CHANGE
TAKE TIME-OUTS WHEN EMOTIONS RUN STRONG

TAKING A NECESSARY time-out can benefit you and, more important, those around you. It should be relatively easy to put into practice, but here are some guidelines to help:

TUNE IN   Only you know how you are feeling when going through stressful or difficult situations. As a result, it is vital that you listen to your inner thoughts and pay close attention to your responses so that you can take appropriate action when necessary. If you start to feel as though you are losing control or that you are becoming overwhelmed with emotion, it is a clear indication that a time-out might be helpful.

TAKE THE RIGHT AMOUNT OF TIME   Take at least ten to fifteen minutes to get away from the situation to be by yourself and alone with your thoughts. If the situation is such that there is nothing you can do to make it better, spend as much time as you need to deal with the emotion. Remember, however, that letting go of the anger is important to moving forward in a productive way.

REENGAGE IN A TIMELY FASHION   If the situation requires resolution, keep your time-out short enough so you can reengage in a timely fashion. This means you don't want too much time to go by; if it does, you may find that issues may never get resolved or, worse, may be swept under the rug. Set a time limit so you can give your attention to the other person or situation within an appropriate time frame.

COMMUNICATE   If taking a time-out is a result of a conflict with or involves someone else, communicate to them your need for space and time to sort out your feelings. Doing so alerts them to the fact that you are upset or dealing with raw emotions, and it also gives them an opportunity to consider reflecting on their own feelings. This increases the likelihood of a more productive dialogue when you return to the discussion or situation.

DO SOMETHING CONSTRUCTIVE   Use your time-out to constructively let off steam. For instance, you might go for a long walk outdoors, which helps you get some fresh air and clear your mind and gives you a new perspective. Meditate to release negative thoughts, stress, or pain. Write in a journal to encourage free-flowing thinking and full expression of your thoughts and emotions. Or call a friend to hash out some of your thoughts and gain perspective.

RESPECT AND RECIPROCATE   If you find you are engaged in a discussion or situation that is visibly upsetting the other individual, offer a mutual time-out. Maybe the other person will realize he needs a time-out on his own, in which case respect his needs and grant him the time-out without any resentment. But if he doesn't, tell him you think it might be helpful if you both stepped away for a short time period to gain perspective and composure. This shows you respect him and can see how upset he is, but also gives him an opportunity to cool off and calm down so, ideally, he can return to the conversation in a more rational and productive frame of mind.

✤ ✤ ✤

BE A LIFELONG LEARNER

Always walk through life as if you have
something new to learn and you will.

—VERNON HOWARD

ALTHOUGH YOU MAY not be in school anymore, remaining a student throughout life can provide a world of benefits to your mind. Our brains are capable of amazing things, yet when we don't use them, we essentially lose them. It behooves us to constantly challenge ourselves by learning new things and developing new skills to keep our minds sharp.

Unlike many of our other organs, the brain has the ability to constantly change—a phenomenon known as "neuroplasticity" or "brain plasticity."[1] Further, new studies show that we are capable of neurogenesis, a process wherein we create new neurons in certain parts of our brain (including within the hippocampus, which is responsible for memory and spatial navigation) throughout our lifetime.[2] These ongoing biological processes mean that we have the power to create physical changes in the cellular structures of the brain, developing new nerve pathways, which can directly result in improved cognitive function, a slowed aging process, and enhanced memory.

DID YOU KNOW?

A study out of London showed that London taxi drivers have a larger hippocampus than London bus drivers. This is due to the constant stimulation of taxi drivers' hippocampus as they form and access complex memories for efficient navigation, compared to the rather repetitive set of routes that bus drivers follow.[3]

Learning and exposing ourselves to new things also provides a constant source of novelty and excitement. And as we develop new skills, acquire new knowledge, and learn new things about ourselves, we gain a huge sense of fulfillment. The mere idea of putting our mind to something and maintaining follow-through gives us a sense of pride, greater purpose, and a feeling of growth—all of which boosts our self-confidence.

✧ ✧ ✧

THE PATH TO CHANGE
LEARN SOMETHING NEW EACH WEEK

IF GOING BACK to school sounds unappealing, don't fret. The kind of learning you will experience with this week's change should be all about you and your interests. Although you will certainly want to challenge yourself and push yourself to try new things, you don't necessarily have to take tests, get good grades, or make the honor roll! The most valuable thing you can do is enjoy new subject matter, spark new thoughts, and have new experiences so you are continually challenged in fun and interesting ways. And you don't necessarily need to learn a whole new skill; it could be as simple as learning a new fact or two about a subject you enjoy.

CHOOSE THINGS YOU WANT TO LEARN   Don't force yourself to learn something you have no interest in, as that will likely make the idea of learning unpalatable. If you are at a loss for where to begin, a great starting point is to think about what you don't know how to do or don't understand but wish you did. For instance, if you've always had an appreciation for sculpture but know very little about the art, you might take a class at a museum on the history of sculpture, or even a sculpture class at a local art school. Or maybe you've admired your friend's cooking ability, so you might benefit from taking a cooking class.

FOCUS ON GROWTH AND NOT MASTERY   To keep learning fun, don't let the idea of perfection or full mastery cloud your ability to enjoy what you learn. Instead, focus on learning for personal fulfillment and growth. This will allow you to enjoy the process and experience much more than if you concern yourself with reaching a specific goal or being the best. And if learning something new feels uncomfortable or strange, that is a good thing! It means you are using your brain in new ways. Try not to get frustrated if something feels unnatural, or you struggle to grasp things at the beginning. Be patient with yourself, just as you would with a child who is learning something for the first time.

GO BROAD AND DEEP   Breadth and depth both have their advantages. Enjoying a diversity of subject matter and learning things that fall outside of your current interests and strengths help you to develop new and more extensive synapses in your brain, and will keep you from getting bored. At the same time, exploring a subject more deeply can extend and strengthen your knowledge base in something for which you have great passion.

KEEP IT CHALLENGING   Make a point of selecting things that aren't really easy for you. For instance, if you're naturally a good writer but struggle with the visual arts, consider taking a painting class or a photography workshop to challenge new areas of your brain—and eye-hand coordination! Resist the urge to keep choosing things at which you are already somewhat skilled.

FUN LEARNING OPPORTUNITIES

+ **ENROLL IN CLASSES:** Many communities, local colleges, and high schools offer adult education programs. Obtain a course catalog and sign up for a class that looks interesting to you.

+ **ATTEND LECTURES:** Schools, hospitals, museums, theaters, bookstores and other retail outlets, as well as other institutions, frequently offer lectures for the local community. Also, check with your local chamber of commerce and civic centers for listings of speakers who may be visiting your area.

+ **LEARN A NEW LANGUAGE:** Studies show that bilingual individuals tend to have greater structural changes in the brain than monolinguals. Speaking multiple languages can improve creativity, problem solving, analytical skills, and other brain processes.

+ **LEARN A VISUAL ART OR CRAFT:** Enjoy a craft or creating something visual. When we use our hands to create or produce something tangible, something that produces physical evidence of the fruits of our labor, we gain a sense of accomplishment and fulfillment.

+ **LEARN TO PLAY AN INSTRUMENT:** Playing a musical instrument activates your brain in a variety of ways and can also help with stress management. If you would like to get serious about an instrument, consider private instruction.

+ **LEARN A NEW PHYSICAL ACTIVITY:** When learning a new physical sport or skill that relies on movement, you use multiple parts of your brain and strengthen other important functions helpful in keeping your mind youthful, such as eye-hand coordination, focus and attention, and fine motor skills.

+ **LOOK FOR SMALL OPPORTUNITIES TOO:** Learning something new each week doesn't have to be overly complicated. It could be as simple as doing a little research on the Internet about a topic in which you have interest.

BE DARING Don't be afraid to learn new things that fall outside of your comfort zone or even may feel a little bit scary. These efforts may prove to be much more rewarding than playing it safe. Remember, learning something new doesn't bind you forever. If you don't enjoy it, you never have to do it again. On the flip side, by taking risks you may discover a whole side of you that you didn't know existed!

USE DIFFERENT LEARNING MODALITIES Some of us learn more easily when we read; others learn better through visuals or pictures. Some learn best by doing activities; others learn better by listening to instructions. Learning via several modalities, however, helps us engage more areas of the brain and solidify what we learn. If you find you learn most easily by watching videos, challenge yourself by learning in a different way, such as reading or attending a lecture.

KEEP USING IT The saying "use it or lose it" holds true with this week's change. "Pruning"—a process whereby certain pathways in the brain are maintained while others are eliminated—occurs when you don't continue to use the things you've learned. To ensure that you retain new information and maintain newly built synapses, keep practicing, rehearsing, and using what you learn.

KEEP A RUNNING LIST Pay attention to your reactions to various situations and conversations. If you notice your interest is piqued or you feel curious about something, add it to a "learn one day" list. Continue referring to this list as you pursue new things to learn.

ADOPT A CURIOUS MINDSET Constantly look for opportunities to learn new things—big and small. The more curious you are about life and the world, the better. Try not to take information at face value; instead, research things more deeply. For instance, if you hear that eating genetically modified organisms (GMOs) is bad for you, dig a bit deeper to understand why.

❖ ❖ ❖

SECOND QUARTER CHECKLIST

WEEKLY CHANGES	IN ACTION?
Week 1: Put Pen to Paper	☐
Week 2: Let the Music Play	☐
Week 3: Show Your Pearly Whites	☐
Week 4: Be a Goal Setter	☐
Week 5: Make Lists	☐
Week 6: Be a Mono-Tasker	☐
Week 7: Forget the Joneses	☐
Week 8: Meditate	☐
Week 9: Kick Indecision	☐
Week 10: Sip Green Tea	☐
Week 11: See the Best in Others	☐
Week 12: Read for Pleasure	☐
Week 13: Give Me a Break	☐
Week 14: Silence Your Inner Critic	☐
Week 15: Go Beyond Your Comfort Zone	☐
Week 16: Get Moving	☐
Week 17: Give Thanks	☐
Week 18: Place Value on Doing	☐
Week 19: Seek Silence	☐
Week 20: Speak Up	☐
Week 21: Put Time in a Box	☐
Week 22: Eat Good Fats	☐
Week 23: Open Your Mind	☐
Week 24: Sleep	☐
Week 25: Give Yourself a Time-Out	☐
Week 26: Be a Lifelong Learner	☐

MINIMIZE
SCREEN TIME

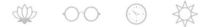

Making yourself available 24/7 does not
create peak performance; recreating the boundaries
that technology has eroded does.

— EDWARD HALLOWELL, M.D., HARVARD MEDICAL SCHOOL

UNTIL RECENTLY, THE television was the main technological device we used to mentally zone out and detach from society. Today, however, we have a plethora of immersive devices to help us do this: computers, smartphones, tablets, *and* TV. Because many of us use mobile devices and computers for work, screen time has become all too pervasive, and screen overload is taking its toll on our mental well-being.

Watching some light television, a few videos on YouTube, or surfing the Internet for a few minutes can be relaxing, but we can quickly fall into "too much of a good thing." Although a small dose of media may be mood enhancing in the short term, regular extended screen time has been shown to have negative long-term effects.

Too much screen time, including television and playing video games, decreases our attention span, ability to concentrate, and cognitive function. In a study conducted by Iowa State University involving both elementary and college-level students, participants who spent more than two hours in front of the television and/or playing video games per day were one-and-a-half to two times more likely to develop attention problems.[1] And the earlier the exposure, the earlier the problems seem to develop.[2]

In regards to computer and mobile device usage, a study conducted by Sarah Thomeé at the University of Gothenburg found that constant use of computers and mobile devices can lead to stress, sleeping disorders, and depression.[3] Mobile devices, specifically, have become ubiquitous; we rarely get a moment without them. Many of us are constantly plugged in, and all of this stimulation causes stress because we lack the downtime we need. Even when we try to relax, we fall victim to constant technological disruptions and the need to be "connected."

Although we feel as if technology keeps us connected, it actually diminishes the quality of our social interactions and means that much less time doing meaningful or rewarding activities. The less time we spend proactively doing things we enjoy, challenging ourselves, or enjoying the company of others in person, the more we run the risk of depression. In a study conducted at the University of Maryland, it was found that unhappy people watch more television, whereas people who describe themselves as "very happy" spend more time reading and socializing. Study coauthor John P. Robinson claims, "TV doesn't really seem to satisfy people over the long haul the way social involvement or reading a newspaper does."[4]

✤ ✤ ✤

THE PATH TO CHANGE
GO ON A SCREEN DIET

BETWEEN PERSONAL USE and work use, we can spend seemingly all day in front of some form of screen. To strike an important balance, limit unnecessary screen time with the following techniques:

REDUCE EXPOSURE Most people are shocked to realize how much screen time they actually spend per day. In a survey conducted by eMarketer, Americans reported spending, on average, almost ten hours per day or over 270 hours per month online, on mobile devices, and watching television.[5] Four and a half hours, specifically, were dedicated to watching television. These numbers add up to about six work weeks per month that could be put to more productive, more life-enhancing use, such as spending time with friends and family, playing with pets, enjoying hobbies, getting exercise, and, of course, reading or learning.

Raise awareness The first step in making this change is to raise your awareness of how much screen time you spend each day. Use the Media Inventory Worksheet in the back of the book to log the hours you spend on various devices for both work and personal use. When done, tally up the hours spent on each device, as well as the total number of hours you spend on all screens per day.

Set limits Most likely, several hours per week are spent on time fillers. Set a goal of how much screen time you'd like to cut out of your week. For instance, let's say you watch four hours a day, or twenty-eight hours a week, of television. Maybe your goal would be to cut back by 50 percent, watching no more than two hours per day or fourteen hours per week. Or maybe you find you spend about one hour per day on Facebook, and your goal is to cut back by 50 percent or limit it to thirty minutes per day. Write these numbers in the last column of the Media Inventory, "Goal."

Implement Each day, tally the number of hours of screen time you spend and continually work toward meeting your goals. If you go over your maximum on one day, try to spend less time in front of a screen the next day.

GET OUT OF THE ZONE   Instead of letting devices distract you, create distractions that take you away from them. For instance, go for a walk without your smartphone. Go to a lecture where electronic devices must be turned off. Or go to a place where you will physically be unable to get reception or a signal.

SAY NO IN COMPANY   When you are in the company of others, make a point of turning off all connected devices. Not only will the other people appreciate your undivided attention, but you will also get much more out of the time you spend with them, making for a more rewarding and fulfilling interaction.

TECHNOLOGY-FREE ZONES AT HOME   Designate certain areas of your home as screen-free zones. This is especially important in the bedroom, as staying clear of devices at least an hour before bedtime is beneficial. As we discuss in Week 24: Sleep, using technology near bedtime keeps your mind wired and unable to settle down for sleep.

ONE AT A TIME   According to a study called "Screens to the nth," conducted by the Interactive Advertising Bureau, a majority of consumers multitask with technology while watching television. Sixty-three percent of respondents reported use of a connected device for at least a few minutes the last time they watched television, with 15 percent using more than one device while watching TV.[6] Try to use only one screen at a time. Further, if you own multiple devices—a smartphone, a tablet, a laptop, and so on, streamline by trading in a couple for one that offers the functionality of both. The fewer screens you have to choose from, the easier it will be to limit your time in front of them.

FORGET DIGITAL AND GO LIVE   When possible, choose to do things in person and without technology. Instead of watching television or a movie, opt for a live performance, such as a play or concert. Instead of playing video games, choose board games or even games that are more physical, such as laser tag or paint ball. Instead of shopping online, go to the store. And, of course, instead of texting, pick up the phone and call your loved one or, better yet, make a date to meet in person.

MAKE IT A FRIENDS-AND-FAMILY THING   Designate one night a week as a technology-free night with your family (or roommates). Not only will this keep your eyes away from the screen, but it will give you a chance to spend some quality time with one another without the distraction of technology.

MAKE SCREEN TIME ACTIVE   The best way to make screen time more productive is to do something active that doesn't require a great deal of focus or concentration. Trade in the chair or couch when watching television; stretch or do yoga instead. Or catch up on the news or your favorite shows during an aerobic workout. Even cleaning the house or doing the laundry makes screen time more productive.

DOWNGRADE YOUR SERVICES   Cancel your cable subscription, down-grade your text and data plans, and limit your internet use. Most popular television shows are accessible on streaming sites. Limiting yourself to selectively watching TV shows through a streaming medium will help you cut back on watching television out of boredom. Cutting back on your data plans will keep you mindful of how much you text and surf the Web on your devices.

MINIMIZE SOCIAL MEDIA PLATFORMS   A huge culprit in the trend of excessive screen time is the time spent on various social media plat-forms. Not only are they generally a waste of time, but they are accessible on every device, keeping us glued to the screen and likely multitasking as well. If you tend to use three or more different social media platforms, downsize to just one or two.

The less time spent in front of a screen, the more you'll see your addic-tion and dependency wane. Look at this as an opportunity to do things you love, to spend time with friends and family, or to dive into a new hobby. That is what life is all about!

✧ ✧ ✧

REWARD YOURSELF

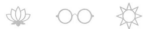

The more you praise and celebrate your life, the more there is in life to celebrate.

—OPRAH WINFREY

MANY OF US are so focused on getting a job done or reaching our goals that we forget to take a step back and actually celebrate our accomplishments. Unfortunately, this behavior deprives us of feeling fulfilled and can also sabotage our motivation to complete future tasks or goals. Self-reward feels good, and it also serves a purpose: you are motivating future hard work, while recognizing the hard work you've already completed.

Goal setting, as we've discussed, is very powerful and important to your happiness. At the same time, it is easy to fall victim to perpetual goal setting, so as soon as we achieve one thing, we immediately turn to accomplishing something else. When we focus so much on the future, it is easy to lose sight of the effort it has taken to get us where we are today. This denies us the happiness that comes with a sense of accomplishment.

Rewarding yourself for completing especially difficult tasks is helpful for inspiring future success: you succeeded in the past and you were rewarded, so you can envision the payoff from taking on new challenges.

The more you reward yourself, the more your mind will associate difficult undertakings with the feel-good feelings of completion. And as you can imagine, rewards for longer-term goals, such as losing thirty pounds or quitting smoking, can make the hard work along the way worthwhile.

DID YOU KNOW?

Self-reward may boost your performance. When we feel loved, valued, or appreciated, we release a hormone called oxytocin. Research has shown that people who work under the influence of this hormone tend to perform better and are more trustworthy.[1]

When we take on challenges, either professionally or personally, and there isn't someone around to praise us, self-reward becomes even more important. When commitment, dedication, and hard work go unappreciated, it takes a toll on our happiness, our ability to cope with stress, and ultimately our productivity and performance. And whether the task at hand is to clean out the garage or to finish a year-end report at work, when your hard work isn't recognized, it eats away at your self-esteem. Self-reward, however, allows you to feel good about your accomplishments, and thus boosts self-confidence and happiness.

✤ ✤ ✤

THE PATH TO CHANGE
CELEBRATE ACCOMPLISHMENTS AND REWARD COMPLETED TASKS

IF REWARDING YOURSELF seems foreign to you, consider the following:

START WITH THE PAST   The first way to celebrate your accomplishments is to acknowledge that you do, indeed, accomplish things. Think back to past achievements. In your Celebrate and Reward Worksheet, list five major accomplishments of which you are proud. Write a couple of sentences about what you did to be successful. In the next section, note three words for how those accomplishments make you feel. Whenever you feel down or discouraged when trying to complete a task or reach a goal, refer to this list to inspire you.

MAKE REWARDS APPROPRIATE   Be mindful not to over-reward or under-reward. If someone were to compliment you incessantly, you'd come to find it insincere or patronizing. On the other hand, if you were never rewarded or if a reward were too trivial, that wouldn't feel very rewarding either. Make rewards appropriate. For instance, if you have been working on a project that required you to give up any social life for a couple of months, plan a night out or a weekend getaway with a group of friends to celebrate your newfound freedom. At the other end of the spectrum, if you finished your work on time and have some downtime, take a break and read, talk with a colleague, or enjoy a treat from the cafeteria.

REWARD YOURSELF ALONG THE WAY   When a goal or project is especially large or lengthy, find ways to reward yourself along the way. If you wait until the very end, you may lose an opportunity to boost your motivation—or, worse, you may quit before finishing your task. Break your larger goal into smaller chunks with applicable milestones so you can create an appropriate reward for each. For instance, if you are writing a novel, reward yourself for each completed chapter.

REWARD IN COMPANY   If a goal took a lot of extra effort, reward yourself by celebrating with others. If you completed a personal goal, invite loved ones, friends, and family. If it was a professional goal you achieved, invite close colleagues to join in the fun. Celebrating with others provides a social and bonding element that boosts the reward's impact even more than if you were to celebrate by yourself. It also solidifies the value and meaning of the accomplishment itself.

REWARD WITH PURPOSE   Rewarding your hard work is meaningful only if you actually value the reward! If you choose uninteresting rewards, they will fall flat. Not only will they not incent you to complete your task or goal, but if you do finish, you run the risk of not feeling very excited about your accomplishment. Make rewards something you really want, something you look forward to experiencing or having, and something that will make you feel amazing when you've earned it.

DID YOU KNOW?

In a 2009 McKinsey survey, respondents felt nonfinancial incentives (praise or commendation, attention from leaders and opportunities for leadership) were more effective than financial incentives (performance-based cash bonuses, pay increases, or stock options) as motivators, with praise or commendation from their immediate manager being the most effective.[2]

REWARD INTRINSICALLY   Most of us are driven by appreciation and recognition. As a matter of fact, studies show that in the workplace, appreciation and recognition go much further than financial incentives when it comes to effectiveness and employee satisfaction.[3] A nonfinancial reward in the workplace could include praise from a manager, attention from leaders, or opportunities to work on highly coveted projects. A nonfinancial reward you could give yourself might include taking a moment to express the pride you feel or the respect you have for your accomplishment. You can vocalize it out loud to yourself, write it in a journal, or share your feelings with a loved one or a friend. Outwardly expressing your satisfaction and excitement for a job well done makes it real and helps build self-esteem.

WAIT   When you complete an especially immense task or achieve something great, give yourself some time to relax and bask in the glory of your success before launching into your next goal or task. This allows you to fully appreciate and enjoy what you've accomplished, but it also gives your mind the break it needs to avoid burnout, to manage stress, and to go full steam on the next project or goal.

CREATE A REWARD JOURNAL Keeping a log of your accomplishments and the respective rewards you enjoyed as a result is a wonderful way to keep your achievements front and center. It also serves as a reminder of the wonderful benefits you reaped from them, and provides you with a sense of empowerment. If you find yourself frustrated or discouraged while working toward a goal, revisit what you accomplished in the past (as well as the effort it took) for some inspiration.

✤ ✤ ✤

SAY YES TO NEW EXPERIENCES

Say Yes and you'll figure it out afterward.
—TINA FEY

WE ARE OFTEN compelled to say no for many reasons. We fear the unknown, we're stuck in our comfort zone, or we don't want to give up control. Although saying no has an important role in life—it allows us to set boundaries, to prioritize, and to manage our time—it can also diminish our ability to be happy when we say it too much. This week's change is to simply put a little more "yes" in your life and open your mind and body to new experiences.

Granted, saying yes too much can lead to a different set of problems, but not saying it enough can keep us stuck in a rut and may even lead to depression. The more we take on new experiences, the more we fight off boredom. When we say no we close off prospects and the potential for something amazing. "Yes," however, opens doors and creates new and exciting opportunities to make life more meaningful and exciting.

In a study conducted by Rich Walker, Ph.D., of Winston-Salem State University, he looked at thirty thousand event memories and more than five hundred diaries, with durations ranging from three months to four years, and found that people who engage in a variety of experiences are more likely to retain positive emotions and minimize negative ones than people who have fewer experiences.

Saying yes builds self-confidence. When we move out of our comfort zone and walk away with a positive experience, we feel more confident about doing new things in the future. And, of course, trying new things helps us grow. It helps us maintain an open-minded perspective and keeps our brain stimulated and exercised, actively creating new pathways. You may even discover that a new experience provides you with an entry into a new hobby or activity or even a career.

Finally, saying yes to new experiences has a social benefit: many experiences involve other people, which feeds our need to be socially connected. And if you are experiencing something with people you don't know, you may even benefit from making new friends and social connections.

✦ ✦ ✦

THE PATH TO CHANGE
BE OPEN TO EXPERIENCING NEW THINGS

SAYING YES TO new experiences can be a really easy change once you get into the right mindset. Try the following to get you there.

STOP TO THINK   Before going with your knee-jerk "no" reaction to new opportunities, pause and take time to assess before giving a definitive answer. Being willing to at least consider new opportunities helps to shift your mindset to one that is more positive and open to new experiences.

UNDERSTAND WHAT'S BEHIND THE "NO"   When "no" feels like an automatic response, assess where the "no" is coming from. Is it based in fear? Is it based in experiences from the past that are clouding your judgment? Is it because the opportunity requires a bit of effort? Is it because the idea makes you feel uncomfortable? If you really think about what is keeping you from doing something, you may find there is no real reason. Unless the new experience will put you in harm's way (physically, mentally, financially, or emotionally), your reason may be just an excuse. Once you can identify whether or not your "no" is for good reason, you can begin to turn your "no" into a "yes." Make "I can't" or "I'm incapable," into "I can" or "Let me try." If you believe something is impossible, try to think of ways it *could be* possible. A positive, can-do attitude strips away the preconceived notions and negative thoughts that tend to hold us back from doing new things.

ATTACH THE EXPERIENCE TO A GOAL   When saying yes is difficult, try seeing an opportunity to attach the new experience to a goal. How might it be helpful in your life? For example, if you are in the process of changing careers, saying yes to a party invitation might give you an opportunity to meet someone in the industry in which you're interested.

SAY YES WITH SOMEONE   If you are unsure of an offer or feel especially uncomfortable about saying yes, invite a friend along for the ride. You'll gain their support and encouragement, but you'll also benefit from sharing the experience, which can bring you closer together.

SAY YES FOR SOMEONE ELSE   If you have control over a decision for a loved one, consider saying yes for him or her. If, for instance, you are a parent and your child has been invited to be part of an exchange program, but you don't want her to go because you're afraid you'll miss her too much, consider a "yes" instead (as long as she will be safe). Giving others an opportunity to experience new things enables them to grow and become more enriched.

BLOCK OUT THE NOISE   Sometimes it isn't our *own* responses that cause us to say no, but rather, someone else's input or perspective. If there are people in your life who tend to run scared of things and to share those fears with you, they may be influencing you or clouding your judgment about trying something new. Whenever possible, shut out the noise of other people's nay-saying or negative attitudes, and focus on your own perspectives and interests.

START SMALL   Start by saying yes to small things to which you would normally say no. For instance, if a friend invites you out for a drink one night and you would rather stay in, say yes instead. Or if you've never had Ethiopian food but your spouse wants to try it, say yes. Once you are comfortable saying yes to smaller things, you may feel more comfortable saying yes to bigger things, such as a new role at work for which you think you're not ready.

MAKE A DAY OF IT   Attempt to say yes for a whole day. Whenever you are approached to do anything, say yes (as long as you remain safe). At the end of the day, take some time to journal how you felt. Did you feel more alive? Did you feel happier? Did you feel scared? Did you feel stronger? Did you feel more self-confident? Were you surprised by something? Try doing this on a regular basis. The more you say yes, even to those things that seem scary, the easier it will become. And the more you enjoy the results of saying yes, the more inclined you'll be to say yes in the future.

✢ ✢ ✢

GET A RUBDOWN

Your body is precious. It is our vehicle
for awakening. Treat it with care.
—**BUDDHA**

THIS WEEK'S CHANGE probably won't seem like a change at all—it is fun, easy, and tremendously rewarding. Quite simply: get a massage.

Although getting a massage may sound luxurious and self-indulgent, it actually offers many mental and physical benefits. Massage has been shown to reduce stress, tension, blood pressure, eyestrain, headaches, and pain. Further, it improves sleep patterns, breathing, relaxation, and the overall mind-body connection. Not only does the average person benefit, but anyone under especially stressful situations benefits significantly as well. In one study, pregnant women received twenty-minute massage therapy sessions twice a week for five weeks. At the end of the study, they reported less anxiety, improved mood, better sleep, and less back pain. Further, dopamine (the happy hormone) levels increased by 25 percent.[1]

Physiologically, there's good reason that massage relieves stress. Research shows that massage therapy lowers cortisol levels (a stress hormone) by an average of 31 percent; it raises levels of dopamine by an average of 31 percent and serotonin by an average of 28 percent—both neurotransmitters important to mood.[2]

Massage has also been linked to improved sleep patterns. Just a few minutes of massage may be enough to do the trick. In a pilot study published in the *Journal of Holistic Nursing*, it was found that participants who received just three minutes of a slow stroke back massage slept thirty-six minutes more than those who didn't.[3]

If you suffer from headaches and migraines, massage can help there too. In a 2006 study, migraine sufferers were put on a thirteen-week massage program. Compared to the control group, massage participants experienced reduced frequency in migraines and improved sleep quality.[4]

✢ ✢ ✢

THE PATH TO CHANGE
ENJOY MASSAGE OFTEN

THERE ARE MANY ways you can enjoy massage regularly. You don't have to get one every week to enjoy the benefits either. Here are some tips to make the most out of this change:

LISTEN TO YOUR BODY   Each of us carries tension in different places in our body. Some hold stress in their necks and shoulders; others may carry it in their lower back. Even though a full-body massage feels good, focusing on the areas that are the tightest can provide the most benefit. Listen to your body and identify where you are most tense, and share this information with your massage therapist (or partner).

TAKE 10   Although a one- to two-hour massage may be ideal, benefiting from massage doesn't have to require a long time commitment; even ten minutes can provide some benefit. Get a foot rub from a spouse or friend, stop for a chair massage in the mall, or install a massaging showerhead in your bathroom so you can enjoy a nightly dose as you get ready for bed.

EXPERIMENT   There are many types of massage to enjoy. Experiment with different kinds to find what you enjoy most and find most relaxing. Although not an exhaustive list, the chart on pages 163–164 provides some of the more common styles to sample.

IT'S ALL IN THE PRESSURE   Massage that uses moderate pressure may be most beneficial. In a 2012 study, fifty-three adults were put on a five-week course of massage. Twenty-nine participants received Swedish massage, which uses moderate pressure, and the other twenty-four received light touch massage. Compared to those individuals who received light touch massage, Swedish massage recipients saw decreased levels of cortisol (stress hormone), increased levels of oxytocin (a "trust hormone"), and increased white blood cell counts.[5] With this in mind, focus on moderate pressure when giving or receiving massage.

RECIPROCITY PAYS

Getting a massage is a wonderful experience, but studies show that *giving a massage* can also provide great benefit. In a 2012 study published in the *Journal of Alternative and Complementary Medicine*, it was found that massage therapists experience a decrease in anxiety levels after performing massage.[6] In another study, elderly retired volunteers were asked to give massage to infants over a three week period. At the end of the study, participants had less anxiety and depression, as well as lower stress hormones.[7]

TAKE A CLASS   Take a massage class to learn how to effectively massage and soothe stress spots. You can use what you learn on yourself or on loved ones who may be in need of a little stress relief. Make it even more fun by taking classes with a friend or partner. Classes are frequently offered at local adult education programs and local massage schools in your area.

MASSAGE DATE NIGHT Instead of going to a movie or out on the town with your partner or friend, dedicate one night a week as massage night. Get a book on various techniques and try them out on each other. Make it especially relaxing by setting a tranquil ambience with gentle music, candles, and soft linens. Turn off all technology devices so you aren't interrupted and can enjoy full relaxation.

LOW-BUDGET OPTIONS Massage doesn't have to be a costly luxury. There are many ways you can enjoy massage on a regular basis and reap the benefits in the process.

Membership programs Over the last several years, massage clinics have been popping up, providing a low-cost, no-frills approach to massage. Membership fees are extremely low, and services are much more economical than you might find at a spa. Further, owning a membership to these outlets provides you with more incentive to get your weekly or monthly dose of a really good massage. A couple of membership-based programs to try: Massage Envy and Elements Massage. Many gyms and fitness clubs offer massage programs as well.

Be a guinea pig Many massage schools provide deep discounts to locals willing to let students learn and practice on them. Often the massages are very good, and at less than half the cost of one at a spa.

Massage gadgets Although a professional massage given by a trained and certified massage therapist is, by far, the most effective way to go, handheld massagers, massage chairs, and foot massagers have come a long way, and make it extremely convenient to relieve tension and stress in the comfort of your own home.

HOUSE CALL If getting to and from a massage or leaving the comforts of your own home diminishes the massage experience, maximize the benefits by having the massage therapist come to you. The American Massage Therapist Association (www.amtamassage.org) provides information on massage therapists in your area.

TYPES OF MASSAGE

TYPE OF MASSAGE	DESCRIPTION
Aromatherapy Massage	Using essential oils, massage is given using a combination of Swedish massage and acupressure/shiatsu. Inhalation of the oils positively affects heart rate, stress levels, blood pressure, breathing, memory, digestion, and the immune system.
Ashiatsu (traditional)	Therapists apply pressure with their feet, knees, and elbows. Treatments include stretching, stimulation, or sedation of acupressure points/meridians, and structural alignment techniques to work muscles, internal organs, and bones.
Craniosacral Therapy (CST)	The therapist applies gentle fingertip pressure to areas from the head to the base of the spine. This releases constrictions in the craniosacral system (the membranes and fluid that protect the brain and spinal cord as well as the attached bones).
Deep Tissue Massage	Focuses on a specific problem area, working on muscle and connective tissue in order to release chronic muscle tension or knots. Although based on Swedish massage, the movements and pressure are generally slower, more intense, and more focused.
Hot Stone Massage	Using strokes from Swedish massage, the therapist uses smooth, heated stones to provide a deep, soothing massage. The therapist may also place stones on specific points along your spine, or in the palms of your hand, or even between your toes.
Manual Lymph Drainage (MLD)	This style of massage involves light, rhythmic strokes that collect and move lymphatic fluid to help detoxify the system. It reduces fluid retention of certain parts of the body, speeds up the healing process, and addresses allergies, headaches, sinusitis, low energy, and infections.

Myofascial Release	Therapists use interactive stretching techniques and varying degrees of pressure to relax connective tissue that surrounds every muscle, organ, and bone. Although this technique can be done alone, many therapists incorporate it into their regular practice.
Reflexology	Reflexology practitioners apply pressure to points and areas on the feet, hands, or ears, believing that these pressure points correspond to different organs and systems in the body and that the applied pressure is beneficial to one's health.
Shiatsu / Acupressure	With "Shi" meaning finger and "atsu" meaning pressure, the main goal of shiatsu is to bring the body back into its natural balance and let nature continue its course. Therapists apply pressure to more than three hundred points all over the body to help regulate or repair the flow of Qi.
Sports Massage	Administered to professional athletes or those regularly involved in sports as a part of their conditioning program, sports massage is often performed before, during, and after athletic events. Although it can include many forms of massage, shiatsu and Swedish are the most common.
Swedish Massage	The most popular type of massage, Swedish massage involves a medium amount of pressure to reach the muscles through vibration, tapping, kneading, stroking, and friction to relax muscles and enhance oxygenation of the blood throughout the circulatory system.
Thai Massage	Thai massage, or Thai yoga massage, is more energizing and rigorous than more classic forms of massage. The person receiving the massage remains clothed. Using his or her hands, knees, legs, and feet, the therapist moves the body into a series of yoga-like stretches.

✦ ✦ ✦

BE CONFIDENT

Without a humble but reasonable confidence in your
own powers you cannot be successful or happy.
—NORMAN VINCENT PEALE

HEALTHY SELF-CONFIDENCE IS one of the most crucial attributes you can
cultivate for greater happiness. It represents your sense of your own
value and worth as a person to yourself, to others in your life, and to the
world around you. Liking, respecting, and accepting yourself as you are
enables you to live the happy, successful life you deserve.

Our life experiences, including our upbringing and all of our subsequent
experiences, whether in school, with friends, or at work, all feed into our
feelings about and perceptions of ourselves. And when those experiences
have been negative, they can do a number on our psyche. For instance, if
you were teased as a child, engaged in unhealthy or emotionally abusive
relationships, or merely felt pressure to be other than yourself, your
self-confidence may have taken a beating.

When confident, we approach life with greater energy and enthusiasm
and are more likely to achieve our goals. We feel more comfortable in
making decisions, and we tend to feel more excited about the future. We

take greater responsibility for our lives, and we trust in ourselves and our abilities to fulfill our dreams. This translates into gaining other people's trust as well, which can be important to getting what we want out of life. At the same time, when things don't go as planned or turn out as we hope, self-confidence enables us to overcome obstacles and feel more capable to deal with life's challenges.

THE EARLIER THE BETTER

Researchers at the University of Melbourne interviewed more than one hundred professional staff in large corporations in Melbourne, New York, and Toronto. They asked participants to describe their level of confidence in primary school, high school, college, and present day. Those individuals who reported higher levels earlier in school earned more money and were promoted more quickly.[1]

When we are confident, we are more comfortable communicating, which makes us more approachable and more attractive to other people. Further, we rely less on the external world for acceptance, and are less likely to fear rejection. We can maintain necessary boundaries with others, allowing us to create happier, healthier relationships.

✦ ✦ ✦

THE PATH TO CHANGE
BUILD GENUINE SELF-CONFIDENCE

IF YOUR SELF-CONFIDENCE could use a boost, there's good news. Self-confidence builds on itself: as you continue to build it, it continues to grow:

START WITHIN   The first step to self-confidence is self-acceptance. There will always be people who don't approve of us or like us, so looking outside ourselves for acceptance may lead to hurt or disappointment, and this approach never fully allows us to achieve the self-confidence we want. Truly accepting yourself as you are, flaws and all, is imperative.

MAINTAIN A POSITIVE ATTITUDE   Those with a positive attitude tend to be happier, more confident, and more comfortable in their own skin. Negativity, on the other hand, eats away at self-confidence. Resist self-defeating habits such as perfectionism, self-criticism, and negative self-talk; instead, focus on positive behaviors.

FOCUS ON YOUR ASSETS   In the Self-Confidence Worksheet in Part III: Tools and Resources, document your strengths, your accomplishments, and your positive qualities. It doesn't matter what they are, as they are yours and yours alone. When it comes to your strengths, take a look at the things you do well naturally. When it comes to your accomplishments, it can be anything you're proud of. Maybe you're proud of your degree, or being a parent, or a recent promotion. And for your positive qualities, think about the type of person you are and the characteristics that make you unique and a good friend, employee, or partner. If you struggle to think of things, ask people you trust for their input.

TAKE CARE OF YOURSELF   Taking pride in yourself has a tremendous impact on your confidence. The more you value and respect your health, your body, and even your appearance, the better you will feel. Although these practices may seem superficial, exercising, eating right, taking pride in the way you dress, and practicing good hygiene all can go very far in boosting self-esteem.

USE CONFIDENT BODY LANGUAGE   Your body language greatly influences how others perceive you and how you see yourself. Making eye contact and using high-power poses (those that are open, take up more space, and exude confidence) sends others a message that you are comfortable with yourself and with connecting with them. Positions to avoid might include those in which your arms or hands are crossed, your shoulders slouch forward, or your head is down. Instead, keep your shoulders back and down, chest forward, arms to your sides, and head up. This makes your interactions easier and also has the power to boost your self-confidence.

DID YOU KNOW?

Research shows that our body language impacts our self-confidence. In her TED Talk "Your Body Language Shapes Who You Are," Amy Cuddy explains that those who use high-power poses, even when they are faking it, feel more confident than those who use low-power poses.[2]

LISTEN TO YOUR INTUITION   It is important to trust your intuition and believe in yourself to take appropriate courses of action. You have the power to create the life you want. Believe in yourself to make it the best possible.

BE YOUR BEST   Anything worth doing is worth doing well. When you know you've done your best and put your best foot forward, it is easier to feel good about yourself. Take responsibility for your actions, and hold yourself accountable. When you can fully rely on yourself, you gain confidence.

KEEP EGO IN CHECK   Humility is by no means a bad thing. Having a healthy self-confidence also means keeping your ego in check, knowing when you don't know something, and being open to learning new things. Continue to seek ways for self-improvement and allow yourself to make mistakes and to learn from them. Finally, don't take self-confidence to an extreme by becoming arrogant. Arrogance is often a mask for deeper issues, including a lack of self-esteem.

✧ ✧ ✧

CULTIVATE CREATIVITY

You can't use up creativity.
The more you use, the more you have.

—MAYA ANGELOU

WHETHER OR NOT you consider yourself artistic or creative, cultivating creativity in your life provides great benefits. In a 2010 review published by the *American Journal of Public Health*, researchers looked at more than one hundred studies about the impact of art on health and healing. What they found was a clear connection between the two. Participating in creative therapies—such as art, performance, writing, and playing music—has been shown to reduce stress, anxiety, distress, depression, and negative emotions. Further, they can improve flow and spontaneity, expression, positive identity, and positive emotions.[1]

Enjoying a creative outlet is a fun yet productive way to give your mind a break from day-to-day responsibilities. When we immerse ourselves in something creative, we become distracted from our stressors, and we walk away from our creative session with a clearer mind and feeling more relaxed. Additionally, experiencing something that isn't a demand or a "have to" enables us to feel recharged and ready to tackle some of the less-appealing tasks in life.

CREATIVE HEALING

In a 2006 study, researchers found that women with cancer who took part in a mindfulness-based art therapy program saw a significant reduction in stress, as well as improvement in their health-related quality of life, including improved sleep.[2] And in a 2012 study conducted by psychologist Denise Sloan, it was found that subjects suffering from post-traumatic stress disorder (PTSD) who participated in a written emotional therapy program showed significant reductions in PTSD symptoms.[3]

Creativity also promotes healthy expression. Singing a song, painting a landscape, or writing a short story can provide the perfect outlet for tapping into some of our deepest feelings and emotions, especially those that may be difficult to face. When we are creative, we give ourselves freedom to explore and express ourselves in a way that is most natural and comfortable to us, which allows for a deeper level of self-awareness.

Expression through creativity also builds confidence and self-esteem: you are in full control of what you do creatively, as opposed to relying on what others think or want. You can experiment without risk and enjoy without judgment. You have full ownership and license to create, build, produce, and generate something in your own way, providing a huge sense of ownership and satisfaction.

Engaging in creative activities can also increase concentration, as it requires focus on a single activity for an extended period of time. When we create, we often reach a state of "flow": a state of performance when we are in a zone of productivity, such that we lose our sense of time passing. We are completely engaged to a point that is nearly meditative.

Studies show that participating in creative activities can keep the mind more resilient and youthful too.[4] Creativity relies on openness and flexibility, both of which have been found to be important in neuroplasticity—a key element to anti-aging in the brain.

Finally, creative engagement gives us the space to be more thoughtful, intuitive, and insightful, which allows us to gain better perspective, new insights, and clarity; all of which are important to optimal decision making.

✢ ✢ ✢

THE PATH TO CHANGE
MAKE TIME TO ENJOY A CREATIVE OUTLET

WE ARE ALL creative individuals, so resist the temptation to dismiss this week's change because you don't think you are creative enough. Cultivating creativity isn't about talent; it is about self-expression and exploration.

SET AND SCHEDULE TIME   Make time to enjoy a creative outlet. Literally block off a period on your calendar so you are more likely to take the break to create. Aim to spend a couple of hours per week, whether you set aside ten to fifteen minutes per day or block off a larger chunk of time on one or two days out of the week. You don't have to finish what you start; just spend time focused on painting, writing, singing, drawing, or anything else that is creative. As you become more and more engaged with the activity, try to work up to thirty to sixty minutes per day.

DESIGNATE A SPACE   Creativity deserves space where you can be free to create as you wish. Designate a place free of distractions or interruptions to be your creative sanctuary. Depending on your creative outlet of choice, design and decorate the space so it inspires, while supporting you with all you need for your creative outlet. If you paint, maybe you require an easel, paint, and paintbrushes. If you sculpt, lay in essential sculpting tools. If you play music, get a music stand and a file cabinet for music. And don't feel limited to indoor spaces; maybe a corner of your garden or a bench in a local park is the perfect creative space.

ENJOY THE PROCESS   The goal of enjoying a creative outlet isn't about the final product or creating a masterpiece. Rather, it is about reaping the benefits of the process and the activity itself. Remember, there is no right or wrong to being creative. Thinking too much about what you create or judging what you produce will stiffen the process and make it stressful. Leave judgment at the door and avoid the need to "correct." Try not to analyze how "good" your products are, but instead let creativity flow without interruption of thought. Let your subconscious take the lead, and avoid rigidity and structure.

CREATE SPONTANEOUSLY   Creative engagement can happen anywhere at any time. Write a poem to a loved one. Doodle during a train ride. Design your own holiday cards. Sketch what you see while on vacation. If you like to draw or write, take a journal or sketchbook with you so you can write or sketch whenever you feel inspired. If you enjoy photography, keep your camera with you, or use your smartphone's camera whenever you can. Look for opportunities in the ordinary to enjoy being creative.

GET INSPIRED   There are so many ways to become inspired, but what inspires one individual may be completely different from what inspires another. Discover what inspires and ignites *your* personal creativity. Maybe spending time in nature does the trick. Play with children to encourage openness and flexibility. Listen to music. Read literature to stimulate your own writing. Watch foreign films to get a new or different perspective. Or hang artwork that awakens your inner artist on the walls of your creative space.

WORK WITH A CREATIVE THERAPIST   If you are dealing with emotional or psychological issues or even illness, consider working with an art therapist, music therapist, or other type of creative therapist who can help you address some of the challenges you face while unlocking your creativity.

OVERCOMING CREATIVE BLOCK

WRITER'S BLOCK or any type of creative block can be frustrating, but committing and not abandoning the time for creativity is important. Even if you feel results are lacking, staying engaged is the goal. Here are a few ways we become blocked and what to do about them:

+ **RIGIDITY:** Staying attached to a certain way of doing things doesn't allow for exploration of new ideas or processes. Remain as flexible and open as possible.

+ **PRECONCEPTIONS:** Thinking too rationally or analytically can give us preconceived ideas of what could happen or what is possible. Artists such as Pablo Picasso and Salvadore Dalí challenge the norm and create art that defies rational thinking. Think outside of the box by avoiding the temptation to create based on what is real or understood. Allow the impractical and even the impossible to inspire you.

+ **PERFECTIONISM:** The pressure to produce something final or perfect causes stress and diminishes pleasure. Focus on having fun, feeling invigorated, and enjoying the activity.

+ **STAYING MAINSTREAM:** It is human nature to want to be understood, accepted, and appreciated by others. Unfortunately, this squelches our ability to break out of the mainstream to produce something extraordinary and unique. Real creative genius doesn't reside in what is popular, but rather in what defies the established and the norm. Create as if no one were watching. Produce something that speaks to you and you alone.

SHARE YOUR CREATIVITY   If you are proud of your creative work, there's no reason not to share. Although you should be able to enjoy your creativity independently, without a need to meet goals or seek approval from others, having an art show or a little concert could be a fun way to celebrate and share your work with others.

TAKE A CLASS   You can certainly be creative on your own, but taking a class to learn about certain techniques of your chosen art form can bring a different level of enjoyment. Taking classes or lessons will challenge you and expose you to new methods that may enhance your practice. Further, taking a class will connect you with others who share similar passions and interests, providing socialization that can be extremely rewarding.

DIVERSIFY   Cultivating creativity in a variety of forms will engage your brain in different ways. There are so many things from which to choose. Although not an exhaustive list, consider trying some of the following:

❖ WRITING

❖ SINGING

❖ DANCING

❖ PAINTING

❖ SCULPTURE

❖ PHOTOGRAPHY

❖ VIDEOGRAPHY

❖ POTTERY

❖ SKETCHING

❖ PLAYING AN INSTRUMENT

❖ SCRAPBOOKING

❖ JEWELRY MAKING

❖ KNITTING

❖ QUILTING

❖ ACTING

❖ FURNITURE MAKING

Also, don't feel tied to any one creative outlet. Explore different ones to engage your brain in different ways.

❖ ❖ ❖

EAT BRAIN-BOOSTING FRUITS AND VEGETABLES

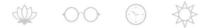

Eat food. Not too much. Mostly plants.

—MICHAEL POLLAN

IT IS WELL documented and accepted that fruit and vegetables are essential to your overall health: they provide important nutrients, vitamins and minerals, antioxidants, and a healthy dose of fiber; but certain varieties are particularly helpful in promoting brain health.

Berries, including blueberries, strawberries, raspberries, blackberries, and black currants, are among the best superfoods or superfruit for your brain. Their deep and rich red and purple pigments are indicative of their concentration levels of antioxidants, including vitamin C, polyphenols, and flavonoids, among others. These phytonutrients are important to anti-aging and fighting free radicals that cause oxidative stress, which has been linked with age-related mental disease such as Alzheimer's and dementia. In a study published in the *Annals of Neurology* in 2012, it was found that women who ate berries more frequently had lower rates of cognitive decline.[1] Further, blueberries have been shown to improve learning capacity and motor skills.[2]

Another brain-boosting fruit rich in pigment is the tomato. Tomatoes are rich in an antioxidant called lycopene. As with most antioxidants, lycopene fights free radical damage, but there's more: lycopene is helpful in maintaining mood by thwarting the formation of inflammatory compounds associated with depression. Tomatoes are also rich in folate—instrumental to good mood, memory retrieval, and mental processing speeds—and magnesium, also important to mood.

DID YOU KNOW?

Although they don't qualify as fruit or vegetables per se, both cocoa and coffee beans can boost brain health too. These plant-based foods are rich in antioxidants. Further, the caffeine in both can improve memory, reaction time, and neuron signaling.[3] And over the long term? A European study published in 2007 found men who drank an average of three cups of coffee a day experienced less mental decline than nondrinkers over a ten-year period.[4]

Dark leafy greens, including spinach and kale, pack a powerful punch for brain health for a variety of reasons. Both spinach and kale are rich in lutein, an antioxidant, which has been shown to protect against cognitive decline. They are also rich in vitamin E, which is important for proper cognitive function and maintaining healthy brain tissue. And, like tomatoes, spinach and kale are rich in vitamin B9 (folate).

Beets and beet juice, also of deep reddish and purple hues, are known to improve focus and concentration and ward off memory loss. They are full of free radical–fighting antioxidants, the B vitamin folate, and natural nitrates. Natural nitrates have been shown to be helpful in increasing blood flow to the brain, which is instrumental to brain function and getting sufficient oxygen to brain cells.[5]

And if you've been avoiding garlic and onions because of dreaded bad breath, you might want to reconsider for the sake of your mental health.

Alliums, which include onion, garlic, and leeks, have been shown to promote proper blood flow to the brain. They are also rich in chromium picolinate, which has been shown to positively affect mood.[6]

✳ ✳ ✳

THE PATH TO CHANGE
INCORPORATE BRAIN-BOOSTING FRUITS AND VEGETABLES INTO YOUR DIET

INCORPORATING BRAIN-BOOSTING FRUIT and vegetables into your diet can be easy and delicious. Consider the following tips:

BERRIES Berries are wonderful fresh, but if they are out of season, frozen or freeze-dried are good options too. Or, if you are motivated, buy in season and freeze for yourself! Clean and de-stem the berries, then spread them on a cookie sheet to freeze. Once they are frozen, store in a BPA-free plastic container or freezer bag. Whenever possible, choose organic to avoid unhealthy pesticides, herbicides, or other chemicals. Some ideas:

Breakfast Berries are a great way to start your day. Add a half cup of berries to unsweetened cereal or oatmeal, a Greek yogurt parfait, or a delicious smoothie. If indulging in French toast, waffles, or pancakes, top them off with berries instead of whipped cream and syrup.

Salad Top dark leafy greens with a mix of strawberries, blueberries, and blackberries.

Snacks Enjoy a cup of berries with a quarter cup of walnuts.

Dessert Skip the cheesecake and go for a healthy berry salad, drizzled with honey.

TOMATOES Tomatoes are extremely versatile. They can be enjoyed virtually anywhere at any time. Swap out toast, potatoes, or hash browns for sliced tomato at breakfast. Enjoy tomatoes in salads, on sandwiches, on pizza, and in pasta. For a quick and easy jolt of lycopene, drink tomato juice (sodium free or low sodium) for a snack.

KALE AND SPINACH Dark leafy greens are pretty versatile as well. The "baby" varieties are smoother in taste and easier to prepare. Try adding spinach or kale to a protein smoothie. Spinach is also a wonderful addition to an omelet. Choose baby kale or baby spinach as your base for salads. It's easy to create wholesome side dishes with these greens: just sauté on high heat with garlic and avocado oil until the leaves are wilted. Squeeze in the juice of half a lemon and toss. And if you are a potato chip fanatic, try baking a batch of kale chips instead.

BEETS Beets may not be the first vegetable you reach for, but they are simple to incorporate into your diet. Here are some tips:

Raw Slice beets up thin and enjoy them with lemon. Another easy way to enjoy is to grate them into a salad or coleslaw.

Roasted To roast beets, preheat your oven to 375°F. Rinse them and trim their tops. Using aluminum foil, wrap them and place them on a rack in the middle of the oven. Roast for about an hour. The beet should feel tender and be easily pierced with the tip of a knife. When they are cooked, take them out of the oven and remove the aluminum foil. Set aside to cool. Once cooled, push the skins off using your fingers (rubber gloves protect your hands from getting stained). If the beet skin doesn't come off easily, put the beets back in the oven for another five or ten minutes. Once the skin is removed, you can slice the beets or chop them. They make a great addition to any salad.

Pickled Pick up a jar of pickled beets or try pickling your own.

Juiced You can either juice your own or purchase beet juice at your grocery store. Consider combining with other vegetable juices, such as carrot or celery, as straight beet juice can be very strong.

SIMPLE BRAIN-BOOSTING SALADS

LONG GONE ARE the days when salad meant iceberg lettuce, carrots, and tomatoes. Salads can incorporate so many flavors, textures, and colors—and when it comes to this change, the more the better. Here's a little inspiration:

+ **RED, WHITE, AND BLUE:** Combine two cups baby kale, a quarter cup of walnuts, a quarter cup of blueberries, a quarter cup of strawberries, and one ounce of feta cheese. Dress with extra-virgin olive oil and balsamic vinegar for a simple and deliciously healthy finish.

+ **TOMATO, ONION, AND AVOCADO:** Chop a half pint of cherry tomatoes, a half avocado, and a quarter red onion. Mix together. Add salt and pepper to taste and squeeze a half lemon over the mixture.

+ **BRAIN-BOOSTING BEET SALAD:** Toss one cup of baby spinach and one cup of arugula with a half cup of beets, a quarter cup of walnuts, and one ounce of goat cheese. Drizzle with avocado oil and sherry wine vinegar to taste.

GARLIC AND ONIONS   Alliums are flavorful and versatile. Garlic and onions are easy adds to side dishes, main dishes, pizza, pasta, soups, and salads. They are also delicious grilled, baked, or roasted on their own: add them to bruschetta, salsas, salad dressings, and sauces. When preparing bread or potatoes, opt for garlic and olive oil instead of butter.

✧ ✧ ✧

GO ALFRESCO

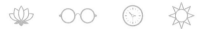

Lethargics are to be laid in the light and exposed to
the rays of the sun (for the disease is gloom).

—ARETAEUS OF CAPPADOCIA, SECOND-CENTURY PHYSICIAN

SPENDING TIME OUTSIDE on a glorious, sunny day elicits a smile and
warms the soul. And there's good reason: both the fresh air and the
sunshine do wonders for our mental well-being. Even so, Americans on
average spend only 10 percent of their time outdoors.[1]

One reason spending time outside has such a profound effect on our
mental health is the increased exposure to the sun. Exposure to light
elevates mood; and, unless you are living in an extremely northern climate,
it's lighter outside during the day than it is inside. Sunlight particularly
plays a huge role in our circadian rhythms, which are important to sleep
patterns. When sunlight hits your eyes, it causes the brain to increase
serotonin—a hormone that produces feelings of happiness and wakeful-
ness especially during daylight hours—and to decrease melatonin—a
hormone that helps you sleep. Additionally, when our skin absorbs
sunlight, vitamin D is synthesized. Proper levels of vitamin D are
extremely important to disease prevention, both physical and mental.
Vitamin D plays a role in the release of important neurotransmitters

(including serotonin), which affect brain function and development.[2] Studies suggest that symptoms of depression, seasonal affective disorder (SAD), and insomnia may stem from insufficient levels of vitamin D.[3]

Spending time outside also means breathing in more fresh air. Although you might think air quality indoors is better, the opposite is often true. Indoor pollutants, such as mold, dust, and pet dander, plus potential radon, benzene, formaldehyde, and toxic gases from cleaners and building materials, all contribute to poor indoor air quality. Studies conducted by the Environmental Protection Agency show indoor pollutant levels are often two to five times higher than outdoor levels, and sometimes more than a hundred times higher. And if you live in a cold climate where homes and office buildings are sealed tight to conserve energy, it can be even worse.[1]

DID YOU KNOW?

In a 2013 study, forty-nine day-shift office workers—twenty-seven in windowless workplaces and twenty-two in workplaces with windows—were evaluated on the effect of natural daylight on sleep quality. Those with windows received 173 percent more natural white light during work hours and slept an average of forty-six minutes more per night.[4]

When outside, we experience improved air quality and also higher oxygen levels. We can live weeks or months without food, and days without water, but only minutes without oxygen. Oxygen is, essentially, food for the brain. Although the brain makes up only about 2 percent of our body weight, it uses 20 percent of the oxygen we breathe. And when oxygen supply is too low, we can experience fatigue, headaches, and depression; diminished focus and concentration; and, over the long term, memory loss.

✤ ✤ ✤

THE PATH TO CHANGE
SPEND MORE TIME OUTSIDE

THIS WEEK'S CHANGE carries double benefits. Spending more time outside will expose you to more fresh air, as well as more natural light.

SET A GOAL   As mentioned, the average American spends 10 percent of her time outdoors. That is 2.4 hours per day or roughly 17 hours per week. Assess how much time you think you spend outdoors, and set a goal to increase your time by an amount you think is realistic. Obviously, there's a need to be inside for certain activities, such as work and sleep, but that still leaves more than 2.4 hours per day that we can dedicate to spending outside.

CIRCADIAN RHYTHM SYNC   Start your day with a brief walk outside. The fresh air will elevate your mood and wake up your mind. And as the sun rises, the light will signal your brain to release serotonin. Do the same at night: enjoy a brief walk outside as the sun sets to get your mind ready for nighttime. Just ten to fifteen minutes can add up to some quality fresh-air time.

COOK AND DINE ALFRESCO   Dining outside is a common practice in Europe. You can find countless restaurants that offer alfresco dining. In the morning, enjoy breakfast out on your patio, porch, or deck. When at work, take your lunch break outside and enjoy the fresh air and sunshine. At home, invest in a good barbecue so you can enjoy cooking and eating outdoors with your family.

WORSHIP THE SUN (SOMETIMES)   An estimated one billion people worldwide are considered vitamin D deficient.[5] Eighty to 90 percent of the vitamin D we get comes from sun exposure. Although too much unprotected sun can increase risk for skin cancer and premature aging, use of sunscreens tend to hinder our ability to manufacture vitamin D. According to the vitamin D council, "large amounts of vitamin D are made in your skin . . . very quickly; around half the time it takes for skin to turn pink and begin to burn." This generally means that fairer-skinned individuals need less time than darker-skinned individuals to synthesize sufficient amounts of vitamin D. Depending on your skin type, consider a short burst of sun exposure sans sunscreen a few times per week (for example, a fair-skinned person might spend ten minutes at a time; a darker-skinned person might need more time). If you plan on spending an extended period of time in the sun, however, make sure to protect your skin with a broad-spectrum sunblock that blocks out both UVA and UVB rays.

PRIORITIZE OUTDOOR ACTIVITIES   When planning activities with friends or family, opt for those that take you outside. There are countless things you can do. Take a walk and explore your hometown or city. During cold winter months, go ice skating, snowshoeing, or skiing. If you live near the ocean or on a lake, go boating, kayaking, or canoeing. If you need more ideas, explore your local parks and recreation department and chamber of commerce for things to do.

GO GREEN   When spending time outside, opt for areas with a lot of trees and greenery. This is especially important if you live in a city where there may be more pollution. The more trees there are, the cleaner and the more oxygenated the air. Breathing clean air makes us feel healthier and more energized.

EXERCISE OUTSIDE   Any type of exercise provides benefits, but exercising outside is even more beneficial. In a study in Australia, it was found that when runners ran outside, they had higher levels of post-exercise endorphins (chemicals associated with a "runner's high") and were less anxious and depressed than when they ran on a treadmill indoors.[6] Whenever possible, take your workout outside: run, walk, roller skate, swim, or bike. If you enjoy exercising with others, head out for a game of badminton, volleyball, or tennis. If you like to strength train, you can do so by going to a park and using your own body weight for resistance

TOP TEN HOUSEPLANTS

NASA CONDUCTED A study in the late 1980s to understand which houseplants are most effective in cleaning air. They looked at fifteen houseplants and their ability to remove three common indoor pollutants: benzene, formaldehyde, and trichloroethylene. The following ten plants were found to be most effective[7]:

+ **AZALEA (*RHODODENDRON SIMSII*):** Does best in cool environment (around 65 degrees) and in indirect sunlight. Filters formaldehyde.

+ **BAMBOO PALM (*CHAMAEDOREA SEFRITZII*):** Place in indirect sunlight. Removes formaldehyde.

+ **CHRYSANTHEMUM (*CHRYSAN-THEIUM MORIFOLIUM*):** Place in direct sunlight. Filters benzene and formaldehyde.

+ **ENGLISH IVY (*HEDERA HELIX*):** Best in cool, moist air. Removes formaldehyde. Poisonous, so keep away from pets and children.

+ **GERBERA DAISY (*GERBERA JAMESONII*):** Requires lots of sunlight. Removes benzene and trichloroethylene.

+ **GOLDEN POTHOS (*SCINDAPSUS AURES*):** Can be placed anywhere in a home. Filters formaldehyde.

+ **VARIEGATED SNAKE PLANT (*SANSEVIERIA TRIFASCIATA "LAURENTII"*):** Doesn't require a lot of maintenance. Filters formaldehyde.

+ **PEACE LILY (*SPATHIPHYLLUM WALLISII*):** Place in a shady spot. Removes benzene and trichloroethylene. Poisonous, so keep out of the reach of children and pets.

+ **RED-EDGE DRACAENA (*DRACAENA MARGINATA*):** Best suited for minimum temperatures of 75 degrees. Removes both benzene and trichloroethylene.

+ **SPIDER PLANT (*CHLOROPHYTUM COMOSUM*):** Low maintenance; produces plantlets that are easy to propagate. Filters formaldehyde.

exercises. If you like taking fitness classes, look for those that take you outside. If your home offers space for it, you can even create an outdoor gym area by using a patio or deck as your workout space.

NEXT BEST THING   The benefits of spending time outside are undeniable. If, however, you live in an extremely cold or northern climate, or you have limited free time to go outside, consider the following.

Supplement If you live north of 34 degrees north latitude (a line that in the United States runs approximately from Los Angeles, California, to Columbia, South Carolina), you likely do not get enough sunlight for sufficient vitamin D production throughout the year. Supplement with vitamin D3 or cholecalciferol (not vitamin D2) to get the boost you need. The Institute of Medicine recommends people up to seventy years of age take 600 IU daily; seventy-one years and older, 800 IU daily; and pregnant or lactating women, 600 IU daily. For infants ages up to one year, an adequate intake (AI) level of 400 IU is recommended. Many experts, however, believe these recommendations are too low and urge adults to supplement with up to 2,000 IUs per day in the winter.

Clean your air naturally Houseplants oxygenate indoor air and clean it and improve indoor air quality by removing harmful volatile organic compounds (VOCs). A study published by NASA suggests you should have one houseplant for every one hundred square feet of living space.[7]

✢ ✢ ✢

SKIP THE
SMALL TALK

Great minds discuss ideas; average minds discuss
events; small minds discuss people.

—ELEANOR ROOSEVELT

HUMANS INSTINCTIVELY WANT to bond with others, and we do so through
conversation. How we converse, however, can have a strong impact on
our happiness.

A study conducted by Dr. Matthias Mehl, a psychologist at the University
of Arizona, found that participants who spent more time engaging in deep
discussions (for example, about feelings, thoughts, or ideas) and less time
engaging in small talk (for example, commenting on the weather) seemed
to be happier. More specifically, small talk made up only 10 percent of
conversations for those who were happiest, while it made up 28.3 percent
or three times as much of those who were unhappiest.[1]

Dr. Mehl explains that human beings search to create meaning in their
lives and do so through connecting with other people. When we engage
in significant, deeper conversations, we create more meaning in our lives
and in our relationships. And research continues to show that stronger,
healthier connections with others contribute directly to our happiness.

✦ ✦ ✦

THE PATH TO CHANGE
ENGAGE IN MORE MEANINGFUL CONVERSATION

ONCE YOU START lessening the small talk and spending more time on big talk, you should see a difference in your happiness and the quality of your relationships. Skip superficial chitchat and participate in more meaningful conversations by trying the following:

CHOOSE TOPICS OF SUBSTANCE   There are some topics you may not feel comfortable discussing, such as politics, but avoid the temptation to speak about topics that lend themselves solely to small talk, such as the weather or the latest hairstyle. Although these can be fun to talk about once in a while, focusing exclusively on these topics keeps conversations at a superficial level. Talk about topics in which you have genuine and deeper interest. For instance, you may be very passionate about the environment, world peace, or foreign affairs. Maybe you like to discuss art, music, philosophy, or religion. Or maybe you thrive on soul-searching conversations in which you can help a friend or loved one work through a problem or dilemma he is facing.

PRIORITIZE TIME WITH THOSE WHO EMBRACE DEPTH   You likely have certain friends, family members, or even colleagues who tend to enjoy talking about deeper topics and are comfortable sharing their thoughts, feelings, and views on various subjects. Make time each week to speak with those individuals so you can regularly engage in meaningful discussions.

PUT A TIME LIMIT ON SMALL TALK   It is unrealistic to think you will *never* make small talk. Clearly, certain situations lend themselves to it: a ride on an elevator, passing a colleague in the hallway, or meeting a stranger for the first time. Although small talk may be unavoidable at times, you can keep it to a bare minimum by setting a reasonable time limit—say, five minutes—on how much you'll discuss superficial topics with someone. Once the limit is reached, either end the conversation or move on to more meaningful topics.

ACTIVELY LISTEN   Take a genuine interest in what others have to say. Deeper conversations require that both parties not only speak but also listen. Avoid interrupting others before they're done speaking or impatiently waiting for them to finish so you can say what's on your mind. Pay attention to what, how, and why they are saying what they're saying. Note their body language and expressions, as these can provide even more information than the words spoken. When others have difficulty communicating their feelings and thoughts, help them by asking questions or offering words or ideas to which they can react. If you're unclear on what they are saying, ask questions to show you're interested while also gaining clarity.

EXPAND YOUR CIRCLE   Join groups that focus on topics that interest you. Some groups where you're likely to find meaningful conversation include book clubs, classes, or community or non-profit groups focused on causes or missions about which you are passionate.

FOCUS ON BEING INTERESTED AND NOT INTERESTING   It is easy to focus on the impression we present to others in the hopes of appearing interesting. Instead of putting your attention on how you come across, however, focus on what the other person is saying. Ask thoughtful questions and probe to get deeper responses from the other person. The more interested you are in what she has to say, the deeper she will go with meaningful details.

GIVE A LITTLE, GET A LITTLE   A deeper conversation requires a level of comfort and trust on the part of both parties. To get others to open up, try opening up first. Share some of your feelings or thoughts on a topic. When you open up to others, it makes them feel comfortable and trusted, prompting them to share in return. Remember, however, not to share too much or talk incessantly about yourself. Share just enough so the other person feels comfortable in sharing a bit with you.

BE THANKFUL   When you find people with whom you enjoy deeper, more meaningful conversation, let them know. A simple "I really enjoy speaking with you" or "I enjoyed our discussion" can make the other person feel more connected to you, paving the way for more conversations in the future. Sharing appreciation also lets them know that you value their openness and candid dialogue.

BE SUPPORTIVE   When some people are nervous or uncomfortable, they use humor to alleviate their own discomfort. This tactic, however, can make the other person feel as though you don't take him seriously or care about what he has to say. In turn, he may be less inclined to share or open up to you in the future. When others share something meaningful with you, avoid resorting to jokes. Be supportive and empathetic when appropriate, and take what they have to say seriously.

✦ ✦ ✦

SEND OUT AN S.O.S.

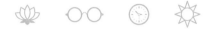

Asking for help does not mean that we are
weak or incompetent. It usually indicates an
advanced level of honesty and intelligence.

— ANNE WILSON SCHAEF

MANY OF US have adopted an attitude that asking for help is a bad thing. We celebrate the individual who manages to "do it all" and is self-sufficient. Those who are successful and who manage to juggle a large number of things, however, tend to know how to ask for help.

Taking on more than we can handle or dealing with difficult challenges by ourselves is not only unhealthy; it is stressful. When we can rely on others, however, we mitigate overwhelm and feelings of isolation, depression, and stress. Asking for help allows you to focus on your strengths instead of shoring up your weaknesses. It allows you to be more productive and efficient because you dedicate your time and energy to those tasks you know how to do and can do well. And when you ask the right people for help, they can accelerate your productivity by accomplishing the things that need to get done in a timely fashion.

Eliciting help can also be instrumental in avoiding procrastination. We tend to put off work or decisions when we don't know what to do or how to do it. When we have the courage to ask for help, we move forward toward completion. And, assuming we ask the right person, we build knowledge and save time by learning new things from those who actually know what they are doing.

Asking for help can provide additional insights and new solutions to problems or challenges. When you solicit help from others, they come to the table with a unique perspective and their own experiences, so they approach problems or challenges differently. They may even have a more efficient or effective way of handling a task, or a solution to a problem that you wouldn't have thought of yourself.

When we are transparent with loved ones, friends, and colleagues about our need for help, it also has the power to strengthen our relationships. It lets others into our world and lets them know we trust them enough to go to them and rely on them. People like to feel needed and want to feel as though they matter. Giving them an opportunity to help you does just that. And when we feel comfortable leaning on them in times of need, it makes them feel comfortable about doing the same. When both people in a relationship can lean on one another in a healthy way, it strengthens the bonds between them.

THE PATH TO CHANGE
ASK FOR HELP WHEN YOU NEED IT

ASKING FOR HELP may feel strange if you aren't used to it. Here are some tips to get over the discomfort and get the help you need and deserve:

BE HONEST Although we'd like to believe we are superhuman, capable of doing everything and doing it well, none of us are good at *everything* or able to *handle everything* on our own. The first step to getting help when you need it is to be honest with yourself. Knowing how much is on your plate, what you are or aren't capable of, and when you can't go it alone is paramount. Thinking you *should* be able to tackle everything by yourself is a self-defeating attitude.

WHEN TO ASK   If you are uncertain about appropriate times to solicit help, consider the following:

Time is tight If you are trying to meet a deadline and you know you are physically or mentally incapable of meeting it by yourself, getting others to help will increase your chances of meeting the deadline and also will help you avoid the physical or mental toll of trying to meet an unrealistic deadline on your own.

You don't know what you are doing If a task requires you learn something new or figure something out, and it is going to take an inordinate amount of time or doesn't draw on one of your core abilities, get help from someone who already knows how to do the task. For instance, if your toilet breaks, but you know very little about plumbing, you are better off hiring a plumber or asking a friend who is handy to fix it than trying to fix it yourself.

Something isn't clear If you yourself are asked to do something and you don't understand the task or don't know how to do it, ask for help or clarification. A simple explanation may be enough to get you moving in the right direction.

Emotional overwhelm We all have times when we feel emotionally incapable of handling something on our own and need to rely on someone or talk with someone to sort things out. Lean on close friends or family members you trust to help you through these overwhelming times.

HOW TO ASK   How you ask for help is crucial in getting past fear and increasing the chance of a positive response. When we ask for help in the wrong way, it can be off-putting to the other person. For instance, if you use pressure or guilt, the person may help, but won't be doing so with genuine willingness, and neither of you will feel very good about the

BANISH FEARS

NOT ASKING FOR HELP often stems from some type of fear. Here are typical reasons people don't ask for help when they should, and advice on how to overcome those fears:

+ **LOOKING WEAK:** Many of us fear looking weak when we ask for help, when in actuality, asking for help is a sign of strength. It makes you more credible to have the self-awareness and confidence to admit when you need help and to know what you can or can't handle on your own. Also, asking for help when you need it avoids embarrassment from not completing things or doing things incorrectly.

+ **REJECTION:** Some of us don't ask for help because we fear the other person will say no or reject us. More often than not, people *want* to help and want to feel needed. If, however, someone does say no, remind yourself it can be for any number of reasons and that, more likely than not, their no isn't personal and has nothing to do with you.

+ **NEEDINESS:** The perception of being needy isn't a result of asking for help; it is a result of how and how often you ask. People get labeled as needy if they ask for help constantly, never appreciate the help they receive, always want more, and never offer help in return. If you are respectful of people's time and show appreciation, looking needy won't be an issue.

+ **INDEBTEDNESS:** Some people fear "owing" people something when they accept their help. If you choose the right people to ask for help, they will be happy to help without the expectation of something in return. That said, always be generous in offering help to others. What goes around comes around.

+ **LOSS OF CONTROL:** When we allow others to help us, it means letting go. If you are a control freak, it can be hard to trust someone else to do the job right. This, however, keeps us stuck. When you are in real need of help, assuming you ask the right person for the job, the likelihood of your doing a better job than the other person is relatively low.

exchange. Further, the other person may not put her full effort in, and you may be disappointed. Or, if you ask the wrong person, you may not get the help you need, wasting your time and leading to more stress. A few things to keep in mind:

In person These days we tend to defer to technology for our communications, which can be convenient but also somewhat cold. When you need a favor or are looking for help, the best way to ask is in person. If you need help from afar, pick up the phone and have a real conversation. The more personal you are, the more likely you are to get a favorable response.

Be clear and direct Whether you just need someone to listen or you want someone to help with a task, don't expect the other person to be a mind reader. It is truly important to be clear, concise, and direct about your expectations so the person has a full understanding of your needs.

Be open Explain why you are seeking help. This gives others a deeper understanding of your circumstances and makes them more inclined to say yes.

Choose the right person Be careful from whom you solicit help. If seeking advice, you'll want an objective party who doesn't have any agendas that conflict with your situation. If you are looking for someone to help with a task, choose someone you feel is competent and that you trust to do a good job. And, of course, to avoid major feelings of indebtedness, choose people who are willing to help without strings attached. If you get the sense that someone is being helpful just because he will be able to get something out of you, he is likely not the right person for the job.

DON'T MICROMANAGE   If you choose people you trust when asking for help, you should trust in them to do the job without micromanaging them. Micromanaging will likely squelch any opportunities to receive their help in the future, and it may negatively affect your relationship.

RECIPROCATE   Just as it is important to feel comfortable asking for help when you need it, you should be helpful to those who need it as well.

This does not mean you should be a doormat and help anyone and everyone in the world, but it does mean that when you can, and within your abilities, you should help others. If you only receive help, but never offer it, you can come off as abusive or self-centered. When you are helpful to others, however, you build stronger connections with people and are letting them know you appreciate them.

BE THANKFUL   Whenever you have received help, show sincere appreciation. Be appreciative when they offer or say yes to help, and thank them when they are done. Go the extra mile by letting them know how their help made a difference to you or made your life easier.

❖ ❖ ❖

GET OUT OF TOWN

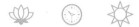

Travel is fatal to prejudice, bigotry, and
narrow-mindedness. . . . Broad, wholesome, charitable
views of men and things cannot be acquired
by vegetating in one little corner of the earth
all one's lifetime.

—MARK TWAIN

THE NEXT TIME you think, "I need a vacation," your brain may be telling you something. Travel, or even time spent away from your everyday routine, provides great opportunities to relax, recharge, and rejuvenate. Whether you escape to a warm tropical destination or venture off to a new city, getting away provides many important benefits.

DID YOU KNOW?

In a 2012 study, 93 percent of American travelers reported they feel happier after a vacation, more than three-quarters (77 percent) believe their health improves after a vacation, and roughly 80 percent believe vacations and the activities enjoyed while on vacation result in greater productivity, energy, and focus.[1]

It probably comes as no surprise that traveling away from everyday life can provide huge stress relief. The break doesn't need to be that long, either, to reap the benefits. In a 2012 survey conducted by Expedia, 88 percent of participants stated they were able to leave stressors of work behind and relax in two days or less when they traveled.[2] Leaving our day-to-day life and environment distances us from problems, allowing us to take a step back and gain new perspective. This new perspective enables clearer and more objective thinking. And if life seems especially stressful, or you feel stuck, frustrated, or bored, taking a break provides an opportunity to refresh the mind and come back with a new sense of motivation and inspiration.

Travel away from home also does wonders for anti-aging. In a 1995 study, Dr. Collette Fabrigoule found regular participation in leisure activities, including travel, is associated with a lower risk of dementia.[3] When presented with new places, new cultures, new foods, and new environments, our brain is forced to reorganize and create new neural pathways to accommodate these new experiences. This neural plasticity promotes enhanced cognitive function and anti-aging of the brain, potentially warding off degenerative disease.

DID YOU KNOW?

On average, Americans who get paid vacations through their employer earn fewer annual vacation days (twelve) than any other industrialized country except South Korea (ten) and Taiwan (ten). Further, they tend to take only ten of the twelve days given. Most Europeans, however, earn twenty-five or more days of vacation each year, and they take all of it.[5]

Travel, especially to new and foreign places, engages all senses. There are new tastes, new sounds, new sights, new smells, and even new textures to experience. Further, it often requires navigating new streets, converting currency, planning and scheduling, translating language, and more challenges that engage many different parts of the brain.

Also, exposure to all of these new experiences opens up your mind to new possibilities. This inspires creativity and strengthens problem-solving skills. The more we venture out of our immediate world, the more open-minded, flexible, confident, and tolerant we become.

Enjoying close relationships is instrumental to our happiness, and when we travel with others, our shared experiences bring us closer together and build stronger bonds. What's more, the memories created can be shared and enjoyed for a lifetime. In a poll conducted by Harris Interactive in December 2012, it was found that 62 percent of adults remember vacations from as early as ages five to ten. Moreover, they found these memories to be more vivid (49 percent) than those memories attributed to school events (34 percent) or birthday celebrations (31 percent).[4]

✢ ✢ ✢

THE PATH TO CHANGE
MAKE TRAVEL A PRIORITY

TRAVEL IS ONE of the most rewarding changes you can incorporate into your life. Here are some tips for making it count.

PRIORITIZE TRAVEL   First and foremost, take the time off that you earn, and when you do, prioritize travel. Although taking a spontaneous day off can be therapeutic, avoid the temptation to make it a "staycation." Aim to dedicate a certain percentage of your time off to travel. And, of course, look for opportunities to use paid holidays for travel as well.

MAKE WEEKENDS COUNT   Travel needn't be of long duration for you to benefit. Even a weekend getaway to a place nearby can provide tremendous value. Aim to get out of your area and explore once a month.

LOW BUDGET COUNTS   Travel doesn't have to be expensive for you to reap benefits either. Camping, backpacking, and traveling cross-country in a car or RV all can provide wonderful experiences and memories for individuals and families and be less expensive to boot. It isn't how much you spend, but rather what you experience during your travels that matters most.

IMMERSE YOURSELF   Try the local food, learn the language and speak with the locals, and visit local favorite hot spots to immerse yourself in the culture of the area you visit. The more you do this, the more you'll challenge your brain in new and interesting ways, opening up your mind and your world. Further, you'll get so much more out of your experience than if you "play it safe" with things you already know or that seem familiar.

ESCAPE TO THE GREAT OUTDOORS   Traveling to places that allow you to explore nature and the great outdoors inspires creativity. Further, facing challenges—hiking difficult trails, dealing with unpredictable situations such as rain during a camping trip, and having little to no communication with the outside world—tests you in ways that help build self-esteem and confidence, problem-solving skills, and flexibility.

OLD SCHOOL NAVIGATION   Avoid the temptation to use GPS when you travel. Although easier, it doesn't engage your brain the way navigating with maps and speaking with locals does. Navigating on your own helps you understand your surroundings better and challenges your brain, which encourages neural plasticity.

VARY IT UP   You may love going to the beach. Or you may prefer to explore Old World European cities. Try mixing things up, however, by traveling to different types of places and taking different types of vacations. This will challenge you in new and exciting ways, making each trip unique, and giving you something different to experience each time you travel.

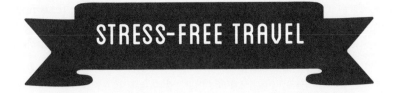

STRESS-FREE TRAVEL

SOME FIND TRAVEL causes more stress than it alleviates. If you are one of these people, ward off the likelihood of stress with some of the following tips:

+ **LISTS:** Maintain lists of things you must remember to pack for your trip for two weeks leading up to your trip. This will help minimize stress due to forgetting something important.

+ **DO YOUR RESEARCH:** Always do research before planning a trip. Speak to friends, colleagues, and relatives about their experiences and recommendations. Surf the Internet for travel forums about the destinations you're considering.

+ **WEATHER:** Stay on top of weather reports, at least five days prior to your trip. They will give you some sense of what to expect. If you'll be flying, and a hurricane, blizzard, or other weather-related emergency is threatening your area or your destination, monitor your airline's website for advisories. Preempt flight cancellations by watching for relaxed change-fee policies on dates of your travel, and take advantage of them by changing your flight ahead of time. Be sure to call hotels and rental car companies with changes, as most won't charge a fee for weather-related emergencies as long as you alert them.

+ **TRAINS, PLANES, AND AUTO-MOBILES:** Minimize connections as much as possible; the more you have, the more likely you'll miss one. Also, when possible, avoid travel on more than one mode of transportation per day.

+ **TRAVEL PROTECTION:** If you fear you may have to cancel or modify a trip, purchase travel protection. This will save you money and stress in the event a change is required.

+ **REMAIN FLEXIBLE:** The more you can maintain a "go with the flow" attitude about travel, the less stressed you'll be. Try not to let the disruptions along the way make you crazy; instead see them as opportunities to bond with your fellow travelers, to see more, or to experience something unanticipated.

GO ALONE   Traveling alone provides opportunities for deep reflection and growth. When we are forced to be on our own, we are given an opening to think about things we often don't confront when we are with others. Further, when we travel alone, it forces us to move out of our comfort zone and do things on our own as opposed to letting someone else do them for us. This boosts confidence and stimulates our brain differently than when we travel with others.

THE MORE THE MERRIER   As much as traveling alone can do a world of good, traveling with others also provides wonderful benefits. It brings people closer together and creates deeper bonds. Look for opportunities to travel, not only with your immediate family, but also with friends, colleagues, and classmates. Ask a colleague you want to get to know better to join you at a conference or to visit a new potential client. Tack on a couple of extra days to see the sights and explore together. Instead of visiting friends in their home environment, plan a weekend getaway together to explore a new city.

✢ ✢ ✢

TAKE A WHIFF

> Nothing is more memorable than a smell.
> One scent can be unexpected, momentary
> and fleeting, yet conjure up a childhood summer
> beside a lake in the mountains.
>
> **—DIANE ACKERMAN**

SCENTS HAVE THE power to conjure up vivid memories. The smell of fresh-cut grass may remind you of playing in the park as a child. A certain woman's fragrance may evoke times with your grandmother. The aroma of apple pie may take you back to family gatherings for the winter holidays. Scents are extremely powerful—so much so that they can affect mood, stress levels, emotions, and memory.

Aromatherapy is the science of using scent to help effect change in our mood, cognitive function, stress levels, and overall health. Essential oils derived from plant materials—such as flowers, leaves, stalks, bark, and roots—are mixed with a carrier such as oil, alcohol, or lotion and then inhaled through the nose, sprayed into the air, or used on the skin.

Essential oils have been used by the Chinese, Egyptian, Indian, Roman and Greek cultures for thousands of years. It wasn't until 1928, however, that French chemist René-Maurice Gattefossé founded the science of aromatherapy. During World War II, French surgeon Jean Valnet continued

Gattefossé's research and used essential oils to treat wounded soldiers. He went on to write extensively about essential oil therapy and in 1964 published *The Art of Aromatherapy*. This publication, along with other research published around the same time by Madame Marguerite Maury, helped to launch aromatherapy in its modern form. The United States seems to have been one of the last countries to adopt the practice, as it wasn't until the 1980s that aromatherapy finally became popular in this country.

DID YOU KNOW?

The olfactory nerve, which is located close to the amygdala and the hippocampus in the brain, is what allows us to smell. The amygdala is responsible for emotion and emotional recall, while the hippocampus is specifically associated with memory. Due to the nerve's proximity to these areas of the brain, many people who experience memory loss also experience a loss in the ability to identify smells. And research has shown that a loss of smell can be one of the first signs of some common neurological disorders, such as Alzheimer's and Parkinson's disease.[1]

Aromatherapy has been shown to be extremely effective in impacting the sympathetic nervous system, which controls the fight-or-flight response and our levels of stress. In 2002, researchers in Japan found that the inhalation of patchouli and rose oil reduced sympathetic nervous activity by 40 percent. Rose oil also reduced levels of the fight-or-flight hormone—adrenaline—by 30 percent. Other oils, however—such as pepper oil, estragon oil, fennel oil, and grapefruit oil—had the opposite effect, raising sympathetic nervous activity by one and a half to two and a half times.[2]

Some essential oils can have an even broader effect than just stress relief. For instance, studies show lavender to be a powerhouse in providing numerous neurological benefits. It assists in reducing stress and anxiety and can also improve mood, reduce aggression, and lower cortisol levels.

Studies also show lavender to be useful in treating insomnia and migraine headaches.[3]

Aromatherapy can help boost memory, concentration, and creativity. In a 2003 study, participants exposed to the odor of rosemary experienced a significant increase in overall quality of memory and secondary memory factors.[4]

Simply enjoying a little aromatherapy can produce wonderful mental health benefits. It is a less invasive, nonpharmacological option for stress management, boosting concentration, and promoting a good night's rest. And what's more, you can enjoy aromatherapy any time and anywhere that it does not bother those around you.

✧ ✧ ✧

THE PATH TO CHANGE
INCORPORATE AROMATHERAPY INTO YOUR LIFE

IT DOESN'T TAKE very much to enjoy the benefits of aromatherapy. To keep your practice safe and effective, consider the following:

PROCEED WITH CAUTION   Always consult your physician before beginning any aromatherapy treatment. Certain groups of people, however, should avoid aromatherapy oils altogether: infants, pregnant women, and the elderly or frail are especially urged not to use aromatherapy. People with preexisting medical conditions, severe allergies, or asthma should seek guidance from their physicians. If you are taking prescription drugs, consult your doctor to ensure there are no contraindications for mixing aromatherapy with prescription use. Finally, certain oils tend to increase photosensitivity. Specifically, avoid citrus oils (such as lemon, orange, mandarin, grapefruit, and lime) prior to sun exposure, especially if you are fair skinned.

SEEK A PROFESSIONAL   To get the most benefit, work with a professional aromatherapist. She will be able to create specific blends appropriate for you and your personal needs. Further, she will take your medical history into consideration. If you are sensitive to allergens or have allergy-prone skin, working with an aromatherapist is strongly recommended. Certification and licensure varies from state to state and country to country. Look for a therapist who is a member of a professional aroma-therapy organization. The National Association for Holistic Aromatherapy (www.naha.org) in the United States is a great resource for locating qualified aromatherapists in your area.

AROMATHERAPY MASSAGE   Boost the effects of massage by enjoying an aromatherapy massage. Many aromatherapists also practice massage and are knowledgeable about which scents will be most appropriate for you and your needs at the time of treatment. (Many massage therapists are also adept at using scents therapeutically too.)

CHOOSE THE REAL THING   If you choose to try aromatherapy on your own, pay close attention to the products you use. Aromatherapy has become so popular that the term "aromatherapy" is used on many personal care products, including body lotions, candles, shampoo, and even makeup. Unfortunately, many of these products contain synthetic fragrances, which do not have the same properties as essential oils. Essential oils are natural and are extracted from the plant. Synthetic fragrances, however, are chemically derived to imitate aromatic scents for personal care products. When purchasing aromatherapy products, choose those that contain the authentic essential oils, as they will provide the greatest benefit. And when possible, opt for cold-pressed oils.

EXPERIMENT   Different essential oils reap different results. And for each of us, different scents appeal more than others. It is important to understand the effects of various essential oils and to work with the ones you enjoy most and that are best suited for the results you want.

Although not an exhaustive list, the following chart provides some information about popular oils and their benefits.

AROMATHERAPY ESSENTIAL OILS

ISSUE ADDRESSED	APPLICABLE OILS
Anger	Jasmine, Orange, Patchouli, Roman Chamomile, Rose, Ylang Ylang
Anxiety	Cedarwood, Frankincense, Geranium, Lavender, Mandarin, Patchouli, Roman Chamomile, Rose, Sandalwood
Depression	Frankincense, Geranium, Grapefruit, Jasmine, Lavender, Lemon, Mandarin, Orange, Roman Chamomile, Rose, Sandalwood, Ylang Ylang
Fatigue	Basil, Black Pepper, Cypress, Frankincense, Ginger, Grapefruit, Jasmine, Lemon, Patchouli, Peppermint, Rosemary, Sandalwood
Happiness	Frankincense, Geranium, Grapefruit, Lemon, Orange, Rose, Sandalwood, Ylang Ylang
Memory and Concentration	Basil, Black Pepper, Cypress, Lemon, Peppermint, Rosemary
Stress Reduction	Frankincense, Geranium, Grapefruit, Jasmine, Lavender, Mandarin, Patchouli, Roman Chamomile, Rose, Sandalwood, Ylang Ylang

WAYS TO ENJOY Essential oils are highly concentrated and should never be applied directly to the skin. They should be diluted with water or mixed with carrier oils, which are vegetable oils derived from the fatty part of a plant, such as the seeds or nuts. The following provides some ways in which to enjoy:

Aromatherapy vapor inhalation Steam inhalation is a popular method of aromatherapy. You can either purchase an aromatherapy facial steamer or use a pot filled with steaming distilled water. Add three to five drops of the essential oil to the steaming water, and place a towel over your head to create a "towel tent" by extending the sides of the towel around the pot. Inhale the aroma for several minutes. Make sure your face is several inches away from the water to avoid burning your skin with the hot steam.

Baths Add a few drops of essential oil(s) to bathwater and blend thoroughly before entering the bath.

Compress Add a few drops of essential oil(s) to a bowl of warm water and stir thoroughly. Soak a washcloth in the water and wring out. Use the washcloth as a compress by applying it to your forehead. You may also use the compress for pain relief (for example, from sore muscles) by placing it on the painful area.

Lotions/creams You can make your own aromatherapy lotion or cream by adding a few drops of essential oil to a fragrance-free lotion base or, for a thicker cream, vegetable butter. Popular vegetable butters used in lotions and creams include cocoa butter and shea butter. Look for those that are cold-pressed for the least processed version.

Massage oil Create your own massage oil by adding a few drops of essential oils to a carrier oil base, such as avocado, sweet almond, jojoba, or olive oil. Again, choose those that are cold-pressed.

✢ ✢ ✢

FACE FEARS

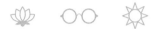

The cave you fear to enter holds the treasure you seek.
—JOSEPH CAMPBELL

ALTHOUGH MANY THINGS can keep us from attaining happiness, fear can maintain a grip on us that can seem downright unshakable. All of us have experienced fear, anxiety, or stress. The more we experience these emotions, however, the less we feel comfortable taking risks, moving forward with goals, and actively pursuing what we want.

Fear is a normal human emotion that comes in two forms: healthy fear and unhealthy fear. Healthy fear protects us from danger and from engaging in inappropriate or harmful activities. It gives us motivation to take action and change our situation for the better. Think of a smoker who is afraid of dying because of lung cancer and, as a result, quits. Or the woman who changes her diet to be healthier when she is told she is prediabetic.

Unhealthy fear, however, is debilitating, keeps us stuck, and cripples us. It sabotages our capacity to be positive, robs us of happiness, and keeps us from living the life we want. It stops us from taking necessary risks when we need to; instead, we spend our time looking for the "safe" way of doing things, which limits our ability to experience anything at all.

Unhealthy fear can be a result of negative past experiences or discomfort with the unknown. Although the feeling is real, it is often has no basis in reality; rather, it stems from what we imagine, without fact or evidence. We tend to envision the worst-case scenario instead of the best case, and this propels us into a state of anxiety.

❖ ❖ ❖

THE PATH TO CHANGE
CONQUER YOUR FEARS

THE BEST WAY to avoid limiting your life as a result of fear is to recognize your personal fears and confront them.

JOURNAL   Journaling about fear helps us release it into the world, making it less scary and dramatic. Look at both current and past fears and use the Fear Worksheet in Part III: Tools and Resources to journal:

Past fear Starting with past fears can be easier than trying to address current fears. Our fears subside with time, enabling us to have a clearer, more rational perspective. Journal about the fears you had in the past, how you felt, if and how you addressed them, and what happened as a result.

Conquered fears Highlight those fears you conquered and use them as examples to cull from your current fears for the future.

Current fear Looking back to the fears you have described, assess which fears still plague you today, as well as any new fears that you know have developed.

WELCOME FEAR   When you feel fear rearing its ugly head, move toward it. Relax your body and your face, and breathe deeply. Welcome opportunities to take on small things that frighten you. As you conquer smaller fears, you'll build your courage and comfort level to take on bigger ones.

REWRITE THE STORY   As mentioned earlier, fear is often an illusion we create, often of the worst-case scenario. When you start to think negatively and imagine overly dramatic or frightening outcomes, stop and rewrite the story. Think about the best possible outcomes and create new stories with positive results.

PUT STORY INTO ACTION   Once you have a more positive story, believe in yourself to put it into play. Don't waste energy on the fear; instead, put energy toward tackling it. Imagine the success, happiness, and thrill you will feel from letting go of the fear and taking charge of your life. When obstacles present themselves, hold yourself accountable and focus on solutions.

REMEMBER YOU'RE NOT ALONE   All of us experience fear, even those who have achieved great things or have done seemingly very scary things. Think of role models or examples of people you admire who you know have conquered their own fears and have done great things as a result.

CREATE A SUPPORT NETWORK   When you face situations that make you especially fearful, lean on others to help you overcome your fear. Friends, family members, and even colleagues can be helpful in getting you unstuck and into a place of action.

✤ ✤ ✤

THIRD QUARTER CHECKLIST

WEEKLY CHANGES	IN ACTION?
Week 1: Put Pen to Paper	☐
Week 2: Let the Music Play	☐
Week 3: Show Your Pearly Whites	☐
Week 4: Be a Goal Setter	☐
Week 5: Make Lists	☐
Week 6: Be a Mono-Tasker	☐
Week 7: Forget the Joneses	☐
Week 8: Meditate	☐
Week 9: Kick Indecision	☐
Week 10: Sip Green Tea	☐
Week 11: See the Best in Others	☐
Week 12: Read for Pleasure	☐
Week 13: Give Me a Break	☐
Week 14: Silence Your Inner Critic	☐
Week 15: Go Beyond Your Comfort Zone	☐
Week 16: Get Moving	☐
Week 17: Give Thanks	☐
Week 18: Place Value on Doing	☐
Week 19: Seek Silence	☐

Week 20: Speak Up ☐

Week 21: Put Time in a Box ☐

Week 22: Eat Good Fats ☐

Week 23: Open Your Mind ☐

Week 24: Sleep ☐

Week 25: Give Yourself a Time-Out ☐

Week 26: Be a Lifelong Learner ☐

Week 27: Minimize Screen Time ☐

Week 28: Reward Yourself ☐

Week 29: Say Yes to New Experiences ☐

Week 30: Get a Rubdown ☐

Week 31: Be Confident ☐

Week 32: Cultivate Creativity ☐

Week 33: Eat Brain-Boosting Fruits ☐
and Vegetables

Week 34: Go Alfresco ☐

Week 35: Skip the Small Talk ☐

Week 36: Send Out an S.O.S. ☐

Week 37: Get Out of Town ☐

Week 38: Take a Whiff ☐

Week 39: Face Fears ☐

PRACTICE DE-STRESSING RITUALS

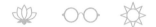

We are what we repeatedly do.
—**ARISTOTLE**

AS WE ALL know, work can be taxing. Even when you love your job, there are undoubtedly very demanding days that can sometimes turn into weeks or months. And although stress from our jobs can be all too pervasive, the commute to and from work can be just as stressful. Enjoying de-stressing rituals before and after work helps minimize the effects of work- and commuting-related stress and provides a mental reprieve from the day-to-day constant pressure.

DID YOU KNOW?

Researchers from Tel Aviv University found that repetitive behavior in general—and especially ritualistic-like behavior—is not only a human phenomenon but also one found in the animal world. They concluded that ritualistic behavior in both humans and animals developed as a way to induce calm and manage stress caused by unpredictability and uncontrollability.[1]

Prework rituals set the tone for the rest of the day and help prepare us for what's to come. In allowing ourselves to enjoy something that is ours and ours alone before the weight of deadlines, the barrage of emails and phone calls, and the long, tedious meetings, we can approach the day with a clear head, a newfound energy, and enthusiasm to tackle whatever comes our way. This positive mindset can do wonders for our productivity, happiness, and general stress levels throughout the workday.

On the other hand, post-work rituals give us an opportunity to wind down and turn off thoughts about work. We signal our brain that work is done and that it is time to decompress and focus on fun, relaxation, family, or whatever personal activities we want to enjoy.

✧ ✧ ✧

THE PATH TO CHANGE
DESIGN PREWORK AND POST-WORK RITUALS

THE BEAUTY OF rituals is that they are yours to design and yours to enjoy. You get to choose what you want to incorporate and how they'll be experienced. Some things to consider:

MAKE THEM EASY AND REWARDING   Whatever you choose to incorporate into your rituals shouldn't be so complicated that you lose interest or motivation to do them. You want to look forward to these rituals, not dread them. Keep things simple to make forming the habit or ritual much easier and more enjoyable. They should incorporate things that feel relaxing and fun, things that make you feel good.

STAY DISCONNECTED   Although listening to music might be a good activity to include in your ritual, resist the temptation to plug into the Internet, your computer, or the television for your rituals. Many of us are highly connected during the workday, which only contributes to stress. It is best to remain unplugged during ritual time.

CREATE A MULTISENSORY EXPERIENCE We experience life through our five senses but, while at work, we tend to overuse our senses of sight and hearing. Balance your senses by incorporating smell, taste, and touch into your rituals. A few ideas:

Smell Burn an energizing scented candle, such as mint or eucalyptus in the morning. At night, burn a calming candle, such as one with lavender.

Taste In the morning, enjoy a cup of joe, green tea, or an energizing breakfast to kick-start your day. After work, wind down with a cup of chamomile tea or a glass of wine.

Touch In the morning, take a cold shower, or incorporate a cold interval during a warm shower for an extra boost of energy. After work, take a warm bath and change into comfortable clothing.

WORKING FROM HOME When you work from home, the lines between personal and professional life become blurred. You need to create rituals that get you out of your home or that take place away from your workspace. This signals the brain that your workday is over and you can return to your home space unencumbered by thoughts of work.

SOME ACTIVITIES TO CONSIDER Your rituals can incorporate anything you want, but some of the following activities may be especially beneficial (some of these are part of the 52 changes in this book):

Journal In the morning, journal about your dreams from the night before or about what you hope to accomplish that day. After work, journal about the day's experiences.

Stretch Whether you enjoy yoga or not, stretching increases flexibility and improves circulation. Stretching is perfect for getting blood flowing in the morning and for releasing tension and promoting deeper relaxation after work.

Meditate Clear your mind in the morning or at night with a five- or ten-minute session of meditation or deep breathing.

Listen to music Before work, listen to music that energizes, inspires, and motivates. After work, listen to tunes that calm, soothe, and relax.

Exercise Exercise in the morning wakes us up, energizes our bodies, increases circulation, and clears our minds. After work, it helps release tension built up during the day. Even if your exercise is a walk to work and a walk home as part of your commute, you'll get the benefits!

Get organized Both in the morning and after work, getting organized can be a wonderful way to decrease stress. Putting things away, doing the dishes, making your bed—all of it helps create order in what can seem like a rather disorderly, hectic life.

✣ ✣ ✣

REACH OUT AND
TOUCH SOMEONE

To touch can be to give life.

—MICHELANGELO

BEFORE WE EVEN emerge from the womb, we rely on the sense of touch. It is how we understand our world while in utero. Babies need to be touched to survive and grow. This need stays with us throughout our lives, providing a whole host of benefits including enhanced communication, stronger relationships, reduced stress, and greater happiness. Not surprisingly, our sense of touch is the sense we hold onto the longest and rely on the most as we age.

DID YOU KNOW?

In a review of research by Tiffany Field, it was found that preterm newborns who received just three fifteen-minute sessions of touch therapy each day for five to ten days gained 21 to 47 percent more weight than those who didn't.[1]

Touch is a powerful stress reducer. When we physically connect with another, we experience a reduction in blood pressure and the stress hormone cortisol. In a study from the University of Virginia, researchers asked participants to lie in an fMRI brain scanner and were told they might receive a mild shock. Participants whose romantic partner held their hand during the scan showed little to no change in brain activity, but those participants who went through the experience alone showed heightened activity in neural regions associated with threat and stress.[2]

Whether we experience a pat on the back, a touch of the arm, or an all-out hug, we experience a feeling of reward in the central nervous system. This promotes feelings of happiness, joy, and love. In a study out of the University of North Carolina, it was found that women who hugged their spouse or partner frequently, even for a mere twenty seconds, exhibited higher levels of oxytocin—a hormone that promotes feelings of love and connection.[3]

Even when words aren't spoken, the use of touch can strengthen relationships and break down barriers between individuals. It is a powerful communication tool. Something as simple as a touch of a hand can help us communicate compassion, love, and reassurance, and demonstrate positive reinforcement, encouragement, and gratitude. And using touch helps us to convey trust and security.

✤ ✤ ✤

THE PATH TO CHANGE
INCREASE PHYSICAL CONTACT WITH OTHERS

USING TOUCH AND being more receptive to touch by others can be extremely beneficial. Some ideas:

TAKE INVENTORY   As with so many of the changes I outline, I encourage you to take inventory of where you stand today. Are you comfortable in making physical contact with others? Do you keep yourself at a "safe distance"? Your culture can have a huge influence on where you stand on this topic. If you are American, Asian, or British, you are likely to keep physical contact to a low murmur. If, however, you are from a Mediterranean culture or South American country, you likely are much more physical. Think about your personal comfort level and how much touch you would like to incorporate.

TOUCH AROUND THE GLOBE

Studies show that our likelihood of touching another human being may be geographically dependent. In a study from the 1960s, Sidney Jourard observed conversations for the same amount of time in different countries. In England, he found two friends didn't touch at all, and in the United States, friends touched twice over an hour. In France, however, subjects touched 110 times per hour, and in Puerto Rico, 180 times per hour.[4]

START SMALL   Depending on where you stand today, move toward making more physical contact with others. If you barely use touch in your relationships, try touching someone's arm or hand while engaging them in a conversation. This simple gesture, if used often enough, can provide great benefits. If you tend to be more comfortable with physical contact, make physical contact throughout your conversations. Always pay attention to the other person's reaction and her body language, however, as you don't want to come off as too aggressive.

SKIP THE WAVE   When greeting people or saying good-bye, skip the wave or handshake and go in for the hug. Granted, you don't want to be inappropriate with work colleagues or in business situations, but if the environment or situation warrants it, by all means enjoy a warm hug.

HOLD HANDS   Whether you are in a romantic relationship or have a family member or friend with whom you are comfortable being close, hold hands, link arms, or put your arm around their shoulder when walking together.

PET YOUR PETS   All species benefit from touch, and when you reach out and make contact, you benefit as well. If you are a pet owner, you *know* cuddling or petting your dog or cat after a long day at work can be extremely relaxing and calming. It turns out there is science behind this: petting your pet can lower blood pressure, improve immune function, and ease pain.[5,6]

CHILDREN AND SENIORS   Enjoy the cuddly nature of children by snuggling with them while reading a story or quietly sharing your day. As we age, we are prone to less and less physical connection with others, so if you have a grandparent or older parent, make a particular effort to be physically affectionate toward them. Don't forget, you reap the rewards as much as they do!

CREATE OPPORTUNITIES   Cuddle with a partner or friend while watching television or reading a book. If you are out at dinner, let your feet touch at the table or, better yet, hold hands on top of the table. There are countless ways to physically connect with others. Be creative! If you look for opportunities, you will most definitely find them.

❖ ❖ ❖

BE HANDS-ON

He who works with his hands is a laborer.

He who works with his hands and
his head is a craftsman.

He who works with his hands and
his head and his heart is an artist.

—FRANCIS OF ASSISI

NOT THAT LONG ago, most people used their hands for their work. In the digital age, however, it is becoming rare to work with our hands to produce physical results. Even designers, artists, and engineers rely on computers to design. Although the technology may save us time, it is robbing us of the mental benefits that come with creating with our hands.

Research shows that producing or tending to things by hand increases our happiness and enhances mental well-being. Dr. Kelly Lambert, Professor and Chair of the Psychology Department of Randolph-Macon College in Virginia, has conducted research in this area and explains that keeping what she calls the "effort-driven rewards circuit" well engaged helps you deal with challenges in the environment around you or in your emotional life more effectively and efficiently. Doing hands-on activities that produce results you can see and touch—such as knitting a scarf, cooking from scratch, or tending a garden—fuels the reward circuit so that it functions optimally.[1]

Dr. Lambert argues that the documented increase in depression among Americans may be directly correlated with the decline of purposeful physical activity. When we work with our hands, it increases the secretion of the neurochemicals dopamine and serotonin, both responsible for generating positive emotions. The less we rely on our hands to complete tasks, the less these neurochemicals will be released. Lambert also explains that working with our hands gives us a greater sense of control over our environment and more connection to the world around us. All of which contributes to a reduction in stress and anxiety and builds resilience against the onset of depression.[2]

When we use our hands, we have tangible evidence of our effort. This provides us with a sense of accomplishment, which builds self-esteem. Further, using our hands encourages a state of flow that engages the subconscious, which leads to spontaneous joy and creative thought.

Manual labor often requires us to slow down. It also tends to rely on process—a process that we develop and go through on our own. And when we can appreciate the process of our work, not just the result, we find a higher level of peace and contentment.

✢ ✢ ✢

THE PATH TO CHANGE
WORK WITH YOUR HANDS

IF YOUR WORK doesn't afford you opportunities to work with your hands, look for opportunities in your personal life. There are many ways to get started:

FEED YOURSELF   Dining out, ordering takeout, and reheating leftovers have become the norm in our culture. Set aside at least one or two nights a week for real cooking. Forget jarred tomato sauce, canned soup, and boxed dinners. Take the time to cook and/or bake from scratch. Enjoy the whole process: looking through recipes and selecting one to try, going to the market, and of course, savoring the results.

CREATE SHELTER   A home improvement project can be extremely rewarding. Plus, you get to live with the fruits of your hard work. No need to build a whole house; try taking on one or two home projects on your own. Unless the work requires a highly skilled trade, avoid the temptation to hire a contractor. Great projects to consider: Repaint your bathroom walls. Put in crown molding to create a feeling of luxury in your bedroom. Replace carpet flooring with wood or tile. Construct build-ins for your living room to create more storage.

LET YOUR GARDEN GROW   Many people find gardening to be extremely therapeutic and rewarding. And there may be good reason: research shows that the bacteria *Mycobacterium vaccae*, found in soil, activates a group of neurons that produce the mood-boosting neurochemical serotonin.[2] When considering what to grow, think about incorporating vegetables, fruit, herbs, or spices.

CREATE, DON'T BUY   Although it may save time to buy a gift or buy something you need, making it not only saves you some money but will make you happier. And if you are gifting someone with your creation, that gift will have greater meaning. Some ideas: Make your own holiday cards. Bake a cake from scratch for a loved one. Knit booties or a hat as a baby gift. Take a photograph of your friends at their wedding and frame it as a gift.

PLAY   Whether you have children or not, there is no reason you can't create with your hands for play. For instance, build a sand castle (take a picture so you can reminisce) instead of sunbathing. Buy some blocks or LEGOs and build something instead of watching television. Finger paint on a rainy day and gift friends with your creations.

✤ ✤ ✤

BE A GURU

If you have knowledge,
let others light their candles at it.
—MARGARET FULLER

IF YOU THINK the word "mentor" doesn't apply to you, think again. Each and every one of your experiences has led you to where you are today. All of your mistakes, your failures, your accomplishments, and your gained knowledge have made you a better and wiser version of yourself. Sharing that wisdom could help another person and benefit you as well.

Studies show that helping others increases happiness for the mentor, in part perhaps because focusing on someone else's problems and issues counters the self-focused nature of anxiety or depression. When we help others in need, we disengage from our own obstacles and become more open and reflective, perhaps gaining new perspective on our own circumstances.[1]

As a mentor, you become influential; a source of inspiration, motivation, and empowerment to another individual. Although this is of huge benefit to the other person, you also benefit by gaining a sense of purpose. When we feel valued and respected, when we feel we are positively influencing others, we feel happier and more confident.

Although mentoring often helps the mentee learn and grow, studies show that mentors learn as well. Through mentoring, you fine-tune interpersonal relationships and leadership, as well as build rapport and trust with others.[2] Mentoring individuals with different backgrounds can open your mind to other cultures, different lives and circumstances, and diversity in general. When you help an individual navigate difficult situations and decisions, you exercise your analytical and problem-solving skills. Mentoring younger individuals helps you stay current and keep a youthful outlook.

DID YOU KNOW?

One-on-one mentoring helps create a happier, more stable society. A study conducted by Public/Private Ventures found that kids mentored through the Big Brothers Big Sisters program were:

+ 46 percent less likely to begin using illegal drugs
+ 27 percent less likely to begin using alcohol
+ 52 percent less likely to skip school
+ 37 percent less likely to skip a class
+ 33 percent less likely to hit someone[3]

Mentoring also provides a social benefit: you build close, meaningful relationships. When you are involved in the lives and experiences of others, it facilitates connections at a deeper level. Often the relationship becomes a two-way street, with mentors finding that they, too, enjoy sharing their own experiences with their mentees.

Finally, mentoring provides an opportunity for self-growth and development. As a mentor, you gain exposure to opportunities, challenges, and rewards you might never experience on your own. You may be challenged in new ways, forced to learn more about yourself, prompted to learn more about the world, and inspired to grow as an individual.

✢ ✢ ✢

THE PATH TO CHANGE
BECOME SOMEONE'S MENTOR

BECOMING A MENTOR doesn't have to be difficult. You can do it formally, through a program, or informally. Things to consider:

ENSURE FOLLOW-THROUGH   First and foremost, you must be reliable as a mentor. The person you mentor will look to you for guidance and support and, of course, your time. When considering mentorship, be mindful of how much time you can dedicate. You don't want to over-promise and underdeliver. Be up-front with your mentee about how much time you can dedicate per week. If you can give him only an hour, make that clear. If you can give more, be sure to block out that time so you don't fall short on your commitment.

RIGHT MINDSET   Having the right mindset is important to the process, and there are certain characteristics that will help you be successful in your mentorship. Although you will personally benefit from mentoring, remember your goal is to help the other person be the best she can be on her own terms. Listen actively and cultivate empathy. Be ready to problem solve and dig deep into challenges she may face. Take genuine interest in her life, interests, and accomplishments, and of course, be ready to support her when she fails. Be encouraging, flexible, and nonjudgmental. In the end, you are a role model, so modeling the right behavior is important.

FIND THE RIGHT OPPORTUNITY   Mentoring should be something you enjoy. If you try to mentor a person in the wrong format or wrong area of your life, you may find it unrewarding. For instance, if you love children, mentoring a child may be very rewarding. However, if you feel drained around children but are passionate about work, you might prefer to mentor a colleague or a college student interested in your industry. Things to consider:

Children When you mentor a child, you have an opportunity to shape a young mind and positively influence that individual for years to come. There are many ways to mentor children and young teens. The Boys and Girls Clubs of America, Big Brothers Big Sisters, and other youth organizations are great places to start. Also, look at public schools in your area for mentoring programs, and see if you can get involved with them.

Religious organization If you are affiliated with a religious group or organization, find out if they have a faith-based mentoring program. If not, consider starting one. Although faith-based mentoring tends to focus on instilling spiritual values and morals, it can also involve mentoring for career, life skills, and family.

At work Mentoring a colleague is a natural opportunity to help your organization and its employees succeed. When you share your experiences and knowledge gained over the years, both new and younger employees can benefit.

Friends or family members Obviously, if you have a friend or a family member in your life looking for guidance or interested in your life experiences, mentoring them can be a wonderful experience for both of you.

College students If you graduated from a college or university, look into mentoring students or recent graduates. See if any have joined your company or are interested in your industry.

BE A MENTEE   To be a good mentor, it is valuable to gain experience on the other side of the equation as a mentee. As a mentee, you will be better prepared to mentor. Remember, a good mentor is well-networked and looks beyond himself to provide help and guidance. Always be on the lookout for opportunities to learn and to build your knowledge and experience from a wide variety of sources, industries, and people.

RESOURCES   If you work for an organization or are part of a community where there isn't a formal mentoring program, consider starting one, or look for opportunities online. There are wonderful organizations and resources that can be of help. Some to consider:

National Mentoring Partnership www.mentoring.org

International Mentoring Association www.mentoring-association.org

National Mentoring Month www.nationalmentoringmonth.org

The Mentor Network www.thementornetwork.com

My Mentor Advisor www.mymentoradvisor.com

REMAIN OPEN TO POSSIBILITIES   A mentee could be anyone, anywhere, at any time. Keep your eyes and ears open for people who may need your help or who could benefit from your knowledge, experience, and guidance. As long as you can offer someone something that is genuinely helpful, there is an opportunity to be a mentor.

✦ ✦ ✦

STREAMLINE
YOUR SPACE

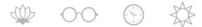

It's not the daily increase but daily decrease. Hack
away at the unessential.

—BRUCE LEE

IT HAPPENS ALL the time. You race throughout your house for twenty
minutes in search of your keys; by the time you find them, you're late to
work. Or you sit at your desk while your mind seemingly goes a mile a
minute, hopping from thought to thought, yet after an hour you have
nothing to show for it. Or maybe you simply forget to do things because
your mind was elsewhere. Clutter, whether physical or mental, has a real
effect on us: it hampers our ability to maintain focus, to be productive,
and to accomplish the things we set out to do.

Studies show that a cluttered environment restricts your ability to focus.
Further, visual distractions make it difficult for our brains to process
information as well as we would if we were to enjoy an uncluttered and
organized environment. This is because physical clutter that we can see
and feel competes for our attention, wears us down, and takes a toll on
our mental resources. When we have a clutter-free environment, however, we are less irritable, stressed, and distracted, and more productive,
focused, and able to process information.[1]

Mental clutter, on the other hand, is a bit less tangible. It stems from countless sources. Our thoughts are abundant. Our have-tos are endless. Our challenges, professionally and personally, occupy our minds constantly. We are inundated with so much information that having a clear, clutter-free mind seems somewhat impossible. Yet making the effort to do so is instrumental to happiness and well-being.

DID YOU KNOW?

Mental clutter may be contributing to aging of your brain. In a study out of Concordia University, researchers found those who struggled to clear irrelevant information from their minds showed a decline in both recall and processing of the working memory.[2]

Removing the clutter, both physically and mentally, will save you time, energy, and frustration, so you can be happier, less stressed, more productive, and more focused.

✧ ✧ ✧

THE PATH TO CHANGE
DECLUTTER YOUR SPACE AND MIND

DECLUTTERING CAN BE therapeutic and rewarding. Follow some of these tips to make it easy and productive:

ENVIRONMENTAL DECLUTTERING   Decluttering your space, whether it is your office, home, or car, will have a tremendous positive effect on your ability to focus and be productive. You'll feel lighter and less stressed.

DISPOSE OF THE UNNECESSARY   If something holds no value to you—meaning it isn't necessary for everyday living, it isn't significant from a personal perspective, or it doesn't enhance your life—let go of it: either give it away, donate it, or throw it out (recycling if possible). Tackle one space at a time, and be sure to finish the decluttering process of that space before moving on to another.

ORGANIZE WHAT YOU DO HAVE   Once you have rid your life of the unnecessary, organize what you still have. Find a place for everything—office supplies, kitchen gadgets, mementos, and photographs. Make use of organizers, drawers, closets, and cabinets to store things that don't need to be readily accessible.

THE JUNK   It is unrealistic to think you will never have *any* clutter. Dedicating a drawer, cabinet, or closet to the junk in your life is completely reasonable. Find a space in which you can put things you don't use on a daily basis but which have a specific purpose or you may use from time to time. For instance, a carryall for your dresser could be perfect for capturing loose change, buttons, and receipts. Or a junk drawer in your office could contain staples, stamps, and coupons. Just be sure to revisit the designated junk space every once in a while to ascertain whether or not you could get rid of something (for example, buttons for a garment you gave away, expired coupons).

GET A CHANGE OF SCENERY   If your environment is especially cluttered and you feel the effects of it, go somewhere else. Take a walk, go to a park, or go for a drive. Or, if you are at work, take your work to a different location that is more serene and minimalist, such as a conference room. Removing yourself from a highly cluttered zone, even temporarily, can be helpful in regaining focus and coming back to the "drawing board" refreshed.

MENTAL DECLUTTERING   Many changes throughout 52 *Small Changes for the Mind* incorporate things that will naturally help declutter your mind. For instance, meditating, being creative, mono-tasking, making lists, and journaling all are beneficial. As a result, the following tips focus on things that aren't covered anywhere else in 52 *Small Changes for the Mind*.

BUILD AWARENESS   When a thought enters your mind, it is either useful or useless. The thoughts that are unessential are just noise and take your mind away from more important things. When a thought enters your mind, observe it and become aware of its level of usefulness. Decide whether it is something to hold onto or not. Ask these questions: Is this important right now? Will it be important in the future? Is this thought beneficial? If your answer to these questions is no, it isn't worth holding onto.

DEAL WITH AVOIDANCE   Our minds can easily fill up with useless thoughts and information when we avoid dealing with things that need our attention. Procrastination, for instance, forces our mind to hold onto thoughts about the project or tasks we are avoiding. Indecision, too, wastes brain space. Tackle the things you have unnecessarily been avoiding or putting off so you can get them done and off your mind.

BANISH UNPRODUCTIVE THOUGHTS   We've talked about negativity and how it impacts you emotionally. Negative thinking also wastes space in your mind. Thoughts that are depressive, negative, and critical should be quieted. Banish from your mind thoughts that are generally unhealthy, including anger, resentment, guilt, regret, worry, and jealousy. These extremely unproductive thoughts take up precious space in our minds that could be given to more productive and useful thoughts.

GET THOUGHTS OUT   Clutter builds up in part because we keep thoughts captive in our heads and don't release them into the world. Writing down or talking through our feelings and emotions, however, enables us to make way for new thoughts. Vent to another person about a challenging situation, or write down all of the tasks and chores you need to accomplish. This allows you to get your thoughts out of your head, releasing your mind from the responsibility of retaining them.

BRAIN DUMP If your thoughts are running rampant and are creating a ton of mental noise, conduct a brain dump. Take five to ten minutes and write down everything that you are thinking at that moment. You may find some of your thoughts are helpful; others, not so much. Or you may find you have the same thoughts playing over and over again in your mind, in slightly different ways. The brain dump will allow you to organize your thoughts in a useful way.

AUTOMATE AND ORGANIZE Find ways to automate repetitive tasks and responsibilities. This eliminates your need to remember these things on an ongoing basis, and ensures that things get done when needed. For instance, pay bills online or have them deducted automatically through a vendor's auto-pay option. Or plug all of the birthdays and anniversaries you need to remember into your calendar, with alerts set to remind you a week before the date. When automation isn't possible, organize your life by planning ahead. Plan out your week's meals, clothes, and chores in advance. The more you can plan, the less you'll rely on your mind to keep track of what needs to be done.

✧ ✧ ✧

BUILD CLOSE RELATIONSHIPS

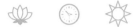

Friendship is like money, easier made than kept.
—SAMUEL BUTLER

THERE'S A SAYING: "If you can count your true friends on one hand, consider yourself lucky." There are many variations to this proverb, but the message is consistent: having dozens or even hundreds of "friends" may seem worth a great deal, but having just a few true, close friends is priceless. In a world where social media has resulted in accruing friends by the hundreds and sometimes thousands, friendship has taken on a whole new meaning. Yet studies continue to show that a few close relationships provide the most benefit to our health and happiness.

Over two thousand years ago, Aristotle shared his philosophy on friendship in Book VIII of his *Nichomachean Ethics*. He categorized relationships into three types: those of utility, those of pleasure, and those of goodness. Friendships of utility are based on mutual need or service, where both people receive some benefit from each other (for example, business partnerships, classmates, or coworkers). Friendships of pleasure are based on finding joy in each other, such as a shared sense of humor, common interests, or even sex. Finally, those of goodness are based on mutual admiration for each other's virtues; these involve deeper connections that go beyond the superficial or the here and now. Friendships in the first two categories tend to be more fleeting, because when conditions under which the relationships formed change, the relationships tend to dissolve. Friendships based on goodness, however, stand the test of time because they are built on a stronger foundation. These tend to be the most rewarding and the most valuable.

Deep, close friendships can be instrumental in reducing stress. Studies show that the presence of a close friend during stressful times can suppress levels of the stress hormone cortisol.[1] Close friends know us best and have a genuine interest in our well-being, so they can calm and soothe us when we are dealing with pain, illness, or stressful situations.

Spending time with close friends also has the power to extend our life, boost brain function, and delay memory loss. In a Harvard study published in 2008, researchers tested more than sixteen thousand subjects and found that social integration protects against memory loss and other cognitive disorders.[2] Another study, published in the *Journal of the International Neuropsychological Society*, claimed that a highly active social life can decrease the risk of Alzheimer's by 70 percent.[3]

DID YOU KNOW?

Having a close friend might save your life. In a 2010 study that looked at data for more than 308,000 individuals, it was found that those with adequate social relationships have a 50 percent greater chance of survival compared to those with poor or insufficient social connections. These findings were comparable to the mortality risks associated with smoking, obesity, and physical inactivity.[4]

When we isolate ourselves, we run the risk of increased depression. In a 2009 study, subjects who weren't socially connected were more likely to suffer from depression and anxiety.[5] Maintaining close relationships, however, brings great joy. Close friends, with whom we can share and confide our feelings and thoughts, provide us with a sense of security. Knowing we have someone to lean on gets us through the more difficult times. Additionally, close friends look to us for support, as well as provide us with feelings of worth and purpose. Both are important to our happiness.

Close relationships entail genuine emotion, sharing of feelings and thoughts, and empathy. There is mutual respect, concern, and support for one another. And when good things happen to one, the other is genuinely happy for the friend, without jealousy or envy attached. True friends trust and are trustworthy; they show forgiveness, enthusiasm, and commitment to one another without any expectations. They share when the chips are down, just as much as when things are going well. True friendship means we love each other in the worst of times, not just the best of times, and accept each other for who we really are.

✤ ✤ ✤

THE PATH TO CHANGE
FOCUS ON MEANINGFUL RELATIONSHIPS

CLOSE RELATIONSHIPS ARE invaluable. They take work and time, however, to grow and strengthen. Whether you are looking to improve old relationships or build new ones that are close, consider the following:

MAKE THE INVESTMENT   Just like a solid marriage, friendships that last take work and effort. If you are especially busy, make dates and schedule time into your calendar for your meaningful relationships. If you can't meet in person, connect through other channels, such as the phone, video chat, or email. If your friend is going through a rough time, be willing to clear your schedule for him so you can be there and support him. Don't take close relationships for granted. Keep promises, be dependable, and stay true to your word. Doing so sends a clear message that you value and respect the other person, and in turn, he will value and respect you.

APPRECIATE THE OLD   Cherish the close relationships you already have. Take the time to appreciate them and spend quality time with those individuals who mean a great deal. Let them know how important they are to you. And don't discount close relationships that are long-distance. These days, it isn't uncommon for close friends to live several time zones away from one another. But out of sight doesn't have to mean out of mind. Make weekly or monthly phone calls or Skype appointments to stay connected, and make an effort to travel to a midway point or to one another's location to enjoy each other in person as often as possible.

INVIGORATE WITH NEW   Although many close friendships start during childhood or adolescence and develop slowly over time, there is no reason you can't cultivate new relationships that are meaningful. A few things to keep in mind: remember that quality is more important than quantity, so choose new friends wisely. Choose those who inspire you to be your best and who are genuinely supportive and nurturing, without any strings attached. Meet new friends who share your interests, as well as your virtues, by getting involved with activities that support your passions and your values. Some ideas: Get involved with a local philan-thropic organization dedicated to a cause for which you are passionate. If you are religious, go regularly to your house of worship. Take a class in a subject you enjoy.

DEAL WITH DIRTY LAUNDRY   As unpleasant as it may be, dealing with differences or uncomfortable situations is an important part of building closeness in a relationship. Conflict should be seen as an opportunity to grow and gain deeper understanding of one another. With that said, focus on constructive methods of conflict resolution by remaining respectful and thoughtful, even when you disagree. Share how you feel, but also listen with genuine interest and concern. Ask questions to be sure you understand what your friend has to say, and summarize and

TENETS OF BEING A GOOD FRIEND

STRONG, CLOSE RELATIONSHIPS that provide the benefits described here require healthy behaviors. Some basic tenets to practice:

+ **STAY POSITIVE.** Negativity, competition, jealousy, and envy are all toxic. Maintain a positive attitude, and be your friends' wholehearted supporter. Compliment them on their good qualities and let them know what you admire about them. Encourage their dreams, and when giving advice or criticism, keep it constructive.

+ **LISTEN.** A good friend actively listens. Be more interested in what your friend has to say than what you want to say. Ask questions and show genuine interest.

+ **BE THE FRIEND YOU WANT TO HAVE.** Be respectful, kind, compassionate, nonjudgmental, thoughtful, and considerate with your close friends. Treat them the way you want to be treated.

+ **BE LOYAL.** Don't be a fair weather friend. When things go bad, it is important to stand by them and let them know you are there for them. When they share private matters or secrets, keep them in confidence and remain supportive.

+ **BE HONEST.** Even when something is difficult to say, it is important to be honest with someone who is close. Clearly, you'll want to choose words carefully to minimize hurt or resentment, but being up front is paramount.

+ **BE GENEROUS.** Give without expectations. How can you make your friend's life better or easier? How can you give more of your time? Try not to think about what you will get in return, but rather, how you can give your friend what she needs.

+ **STAY CLEAR OF TOXIC BEHAVIORS.** When forming new friendships, attempt to stay clear of those who are demanding, negative, or critical, or who don't respect boundaries. Avoid people who drain your energy, and focus on building relationships with those who give you energy.

share what you've heard. Avoid criticism and defensiveness. Share responsibility in making things right, and when you are wrong, be open and honest in admitting to it. If things go poorly when dealing with conflict, take a break, but be sure to return to the discussion in a timely fashion so the conflict doesn't get swept under the rug or dismissed.

BE FORGIVING   We all have moments when we disappoint or are too busy. When close friends seem to have less time for us, understand their need for space. Maybe they are overwhelmed at work or are going through a rough patch personally. Similarly, if you need space, communicate that to friends and loved ones. Also, don't impose unrealistic expectations on your relationships. All of us are human. We forget birthdays or other important events. We might forget to write a thank-you note or a Christmas card. And sometimes a close friend may even hurt us. If warranted, speak to your friend about how he's hurt you, and forgive him when he sincerely apologizes, so you can let go and move on. And if you ever do something wrong or hurtful, admit to your transgressions, be genuinely apologetic, and ask for forgiveness. Hanging onto past mistakes and disappointments will only erode the friendship.

RESPECT DIFFERENCES   Our close friends may have distasteful qualities or characteristics or opinions that differ from ours. If you value the friendship, acknowledge your friend's shortcomings, while accepting her for who she is and respecting her choices. And, of course, if your friend sees things differently or is different, but you believe the friendship is worth the investment, look for common ground on which to keep the friendship strong. Different doesn't always equal "bad."

SHARE   This may seem like common sense, but close relationships are built on sharing through communication. When talking with a close friend or family member, resist the temptation to constantly discuss the same topic (for example, troubles with romantic relationships or work) or superficial topics. Instead, look to foster communication in multiple areas of your life and in areas that are meaningful to you. Expose yourself a bit by discussing your fears, passions, regrets (if you have any), and philosophies. Consider conversing about controversial topics such as politics, religion, and world issues. The more you share with the other person, the more inclined he will be to open himself up to you. And, when he does, be sure to listen openly to what he has to say. The deeper the topics you discuss, the closer you'll become, and the more you'll learn and grow.

BUILD IN GOOD   Close relationships require mutual support during tough times, but it is equally important to have fun and enjoy positive moments. Shared positive experiences are opportunities to bring you closer together and give you memories to reminisce about for years to come. Keep things fresh by exploring together and trying new things. Also, celebrate important moments with each other. Everything from job promotions to birthdays to major life events should be celebrated.

✣ ✣ ✣

SCHEDULE TO-DOS

He who fails to plan, plans to fail.

—WINSTON CHURCHILL

SO OFTEN IT seems as though the days fly by and we are left wondering, "Where did the time go?" Life can be hectic. So much so that when we don't manage our time and schedule what needs to get done, things slip through the cracks. Scheduling your day, however, reduces stress, boosts productivity, and allows you to more efficiently accomplish what you want to.

Whether you want to get to the gym three days a week, finish a project, or tend to errands, scheduling activities and tasks in a visual planner increases your chances of doing them. Scheduling gives us a road map to navigate the day. When we take time to plan, it minimizes unnecessary stress of forgetting something important. And because we are forced to think through realistic time frames for each activity and block off appropriate times for each, we reduce the likelihood of not doing something because time "got away from us."

Keeping a planner helps eliminate wasted time and energy. It enables us to lump together similar tasks or those that need to occur in the same location, reducing downtime and travel time that can easily add up to many wasted hours. A schedule also frees up your mental energy because it relieves you of the responsibility of having to remember everything that needs to get done. And scheduling allows you to see the big picture so you are better equipped to handle unexpected changes or situations that arise. You can more easily see what will be impacted and address those situations appropriately.

Following a schedule for the day allows you to maximize productivity. When you have an hour-by-hour plan, you avoid getting distracted or sidetracked with other things that are less important. Further, you reduce the likelihood of letting an activity go on for too long. For instance, meetings can be a huge time waster, running much longer than necessary. If you call a meeting and keep to a schedule, however, you eliminate the possibility of going into overtime, because your schedule dictates when the meeting must end. Scheduling also helps you overcome procrastination. When you have a scheduled task, the visual reminder solidifies its importance and increases your sense of accountability. It also gives you a handy reference so you don't waste time thinking about what you need to do next.

DID YOU KNOW?

In an opinion poll by Salary.com, office workers ranked meetings as the number one time waster.[1] Further, in another poll, by the Centre for Economics & Business Research, office workers stated that on average they spend four hours a week in meetings, and that more than half of that time is wasted.[2]

Finally, you remove the stress of possibly double-booking yourself. When obligations are effectively laid out in a planner, you'll know your availability more clearly and be able to make (and keep) commitments more confidently. You'll be more reliable and dependable overall.

✦ ✦ ✦

THE PATH TO CHANGE
SCHEDULE ALL OF YOUR ACTIVITIES IN A PLANNER

BOOST PRODUCTIVITY AND save time by maintaining a schedule each day. Here are some tips to make your planner effective:

MEDIUM   Choose a planner that is going to be easy for you to maintain. There are tons to choose from, including calendars, hard-copy journals, and organizers, and, of course, all of the available digital software and products. Choose whatever seems most intuitive for you—whatever allows you to easily enter and access information whenever you need it.

WHAT TO INCLUDE   If you find yourself saying, "I didn't have time to go to the gym today," that indicates it should be scheduled into your calendar. When we block off time in our day for a specific activity, we are much more likely to do it. Include everything in your planner that you deem important. This can include meetings with people, head-down uninterrupted work time, phone calls, lunch or dinner dates, concerts, going to the gym, grocery shopping, downtime, or whatever else you want to make sure happens that day. Additionally, look way into the future when scheduling. Write in important deadlines, milestones, birthdays, anniversaries, and anything else that should be acknowledged or celebrated.

BE SPECIFIC   Be thorough when writing to-dos into your schedule. Include as much information as possible, including the task, the people with whom you're meeting, the location of the meeting or activity, and any phone numbers or other logistical information you need. For instance, if you have a conference call, include the dial-in information and pass codes in your schedule to avoid wasted time and unnecessary stress from needing to search for the information at the last minute. Being specific will make it easier to perform your task without any hiccups.

INCLUDE NON-TASK TIME   To-dos may require preparation, travel, or other logistics before and/or after. For instance, if you have a date for lunch across town, you may need fifteen minutes of travel time, both to and from your lunch meeting. Or if you are going to the gym, you may need time to get to the gym and change, and shower and change afterward, in addition to the workout itself. Be sure to account for this when blocking off time in your schedule.

DON'T SCHEDULE TOO TIGHTLY   You will always have unforeseen delays, discussions, calls, or interruptions that disrupt your schedule. To avoid getting backed up or missing important meetings or activities, don't overcrowd your schedule. Build in a cushion of a half hour a few times each day to give yourself padding between events. This also gives you flexibility to rearrange your schedule, if need be.

BE CONSISTENT   As soon as you know of an activity or task, put it in your planner. This will prevent forgetting to enter it later on. At the beginning of the week, review your schedule for the week ahead so you know what you have coming up that week. Every morning, review what you have scheduled that day, and every evening, review what you accomplished and look ahead to the next day. Keeping mentally connected to your schedule will help you avoid forgetting things, scheduling things too close together, or being unprepared for meetings or other activities that may require work or preparation beforehand.

❖ ❖ ❖

PLAY

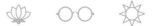

You can discover more about a person in an hour of
play than in a year of conversation.

—PLATO

WHEN LIFE IS packed with work, have-tos, and obligations, it is easy to
forget to have fun along the way. Building fun into your life, even at work,
is essential to happiness, and it has the power to help you manage stress,
strengthen relationships, and boost creativity and productivity levels.

PLAY LEADS TO SUCCESS

While conducting research on murderers, Dr. Stuart Brown,
founder of the National Institute for Play, found a common
link among killers: they lacked play during their childhood.
Since then, Dr. Brown has interviewed thousands of
individuals, including artists, businessmen and -women,
Nobel Prize winners, and, yes, prisoners, to capture their
"play histories." Interestingly, he has found a strong
correlation between play and success.

In his book, *Play: How It Shapes the Brain, Opens the Imagination, and Invigorates the Soul*, Dr. Brown discusses how play impacts our life. Clearly, when we are doing something we enjoy, it makes us happy. Engaging in play, however, also helps us transform negative thoughts and feelings into those that are more positive, constructive, and optimistic. Stressors, dilemmas, and challenges become secondary when we are having fun; our minds get to relax and take a break, so they can come back to problems with new perspective and restored energy.

When it comes to work, Dr. Brown claims that allowing employees to engage in something playful leads to increased productivity and motivation and may improve concentration and perseverance. He states there is evidence that engaging in play can open up new neural connections in the brain, boosting creativity in the process. Also, when we are having fun and involved in play, we lose some of our inhibitions and stop censoring our thoughts. This understanding has led some forward-thinking corporations, such as Google, to incorporate play into the workplace.

✦ ✦ ✦

THE PATH TO CHANGE
INCORPORATE PLAY INTO ALL ASPECTS OF LIFE

WHETHER YOU ARE spending time with family or friends or at work with colleagues, build fun and play into each day. A little play can go a long way!

TAKE AN ASSESSMENT   For most adults, our experience with play generally occurred when we were children. Children tend to be spontaneous, uninhibited, and extremely imaginative. If, as an adult, you struggle to find things that feel playful, revisiting your childhood might help. Think about what qualified as fun or playtime when you were younger. To get started, take the Play Assessment in Part III: Tools and Resources.

It doesn't take much to get in a little playtime. Simple activities such as throwing a Frisbee, playing a game of kickball, or playing hide and seek with children for half an hour can bring great joy to your rather ordinary day. On weekend evenings, instead of going out on the town, stay in and play a rousing game of Pictionary or charades with family or friends. Even spending some time joking around can be an easy way to get a little play into your day.

BE WELL-ROUNDED   Don't save play only for the weekend. Remember that play is beneficial in all aspects of life. Look for ways to have more fun or play at work, when running errands, when cooking and cleaning, or when driving (just be sure to choose an activity that allows you to keep your eyes on the road and drive defensively, such as singing with the radio). The more opportunities you give yourself to let loose a little bit and enjoy the moment of spontaneous play, the more you'll benefit.

FORGET [FILL IN THE BLANK]   There are many reasons to be playful, but many of us seem to find even more reasons not to be. Forget whatever it is that holds you back. Forget following rules (as long as you are safe, not harming anyone, and not breaking the law). Forget what you're "supposed to do." Forget logic. Forget needing to be busy. Forget what people will think of you. Forget doing the proper or expected thing. And forget fear. Just do something that makes you happy and that feels fun.

START SIMPLE   The act of being playful or silly itself can count as fun. Tell a joke. Do a funny impression of someone you know (with the best of intentions, of course!). Do a goofy dance in your office. Do something that makes you smile. Even if it is just for a few minutes, it could make a difference in lifting spirits, unlocking creativity, or boosting productivity.

USE FUN AS A CATALYST   In Dr. Brown's book, *Play*, he discusses play as a catalyst that can go a long way toward boosting productivity and happiness. If you feel unmotivated, are at a standstill making a decision, or have difficulty completing work or a task, do something fun that gives you the mental break you need, while also potentially sparking new thoughts or ideas about the problem you are facing.

BE PLAYFUL WITH OTHERS   When we enjoy playful activities with others, it brings us closer to them. Playing with friends and family is a great way to build memories and stronger bonds. Find ways to have fun with colleagues as well. More than likely, the more fun you have with people at work, the better you will work together. And of course, whenever possible, choose to enjoy time with fun and playful people—children and pets included. If you struggle to release your own playfulness, their playful energy can be contagious and help you loosen up.

MAKE IT REAL   When it comes to fun, "fake it until you make it" doesn't really apply. There is a difference between having genuine fun and feigning it. Real fun is going to feel good, before, during, and after you have it, and it will feel good for all parties involved. Real fun inspires and motivates. Real fun leaves you wanting more, not less. If the activities you partake in don't leave you feeling this way, you may be engaging in faux fun.

✣ ✣ ✣

SET INTENTIONS

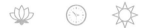

Our intention creates our reality.

—WAYNE DYER

SETTING INTENTIONS CONNECTS us to our values, our aspirations, our character, and our beliefs. This can bring greater happiness and a sense of peace to our life. For instance, your intention may be to be generous, to be supportive of others, to be authentic, or to listen. Intentions come from your soul and revolve around your core being.

All of us are works in progress, and so are our lives. We are always shaping and navigating life as we respond to changing circumstances. When we are tested or confronted with challenges, it is easy to lose sight of the bigger picture. In consciously setting intentions, we give ourselves the space we need to take a step back and remind ourselves—through the good and the bad, the ups and the downs—of the things we care about most and the type of person we want to be. The more we can stay connected to these deeper qualities that make us who we are, the happier we will be.

Research by neuroscientist Alvaro Pascual-Leone of the Harvard Medical School shows that when we merely think about something, it can alter the physical structure and function of the brain. With two groups of participants, one was asked to learn a five-finger piano exercise and practice it for two hours every day for five days; the second group was asked to *think* about practicing the exercise. When both groups were compared, both showed changes in the motor cortex of the brain. His findings imply that the intention of doing something can have as much influence in rewiring the brain as actually doing it.[1]

Setting intentions shapes our decision making and guides our thoughts and actions. We can feel confident that, regardless of the outcome, our actions are in concert with what we believe and value. This enables us to feel more at peace with our decisions and ourselves.

✦ ✦ ✦

THE PATH TO CHANGE
PRACTICE SETTING DAILY INTENTIONS

SETTING INTENTIONS CAN be useful in almost all aspects of life. Some thoughts to consider:

START THE DAY RIGHT   The thoughts and choices you make from the minute you wake up have a huge influence on the rest of the day. For instance, if you are trying to lose weight and you eat a healthy breakfast and go to the gym in the morning, you are more likely to make healthy choices from then on. On the other hand, if you skip the gym and eat an unhealthy breakfast, or skip breakfast altogether, you are likely setting yourself up to make poor decisions for the rest of the day. This holds true for your thoughts as well. When your begin your day with positive thoughts, it has a ripple effect throughout the day. Although you can set intentions at any time, beginning each day with an intention sets the tone for the hours to come.

FIVE STEPS FOR HARNESSING THE POWER OF INTENTION

In Deepak Chopra's *The Seven Spiritual Laws of Success*, he outlines five steps for harnessing the power of intention:

✤ Start in the "gap"—a state of pure awareness often found during meditation
✤ Release your intention once you've made it (stop thinking about it)
✤ Remain centered by refusing to be influenced by others' doubts or criticisms
✤ Detach from the outcome or result and welcome uncertainty
✤ Trust in letting the Universe handle the details[2]

KEEP HAPPINESS AND PEACE IN MIND   Whatever your intentions, they should embody your higher self. Don't focus on materialistic things or specific results, but rather the intention of exemplifying characteristics that will lead you to a state of greater happiness. Your intentions should truly reflect who you want to be at your very core.

STAY IN THE PRESENT   Unlike goals, your intentions should represent the here and now. Don't look too far into the future. Focus on your desires in the present moment. For example, if you are visiting a family member who is ill, your intention might be to be supportive and nurturing. If you will be seeing a friend who needs guidance, your intention could be to listen without judgment. If you are a parent and will be spending the day with your child, your intention may be to let go, act like a kid, and have fun.

BE AUTHENTIC   When setting an intention, be true to yourself and your own desires. Think about who you are, what you really want, and what you expect of yourself. Don't defer to what others want or expect of you.

KEEP A JOURNAL   Whenever you set an intention, write it down in a journal. Documenting it makes it more real than when we keep it in our thoughts alone. At the end of the day, journal whether or not you were successful in fulfilling your intent. If you weren't, write down what you could have done differently to fulfill it. Every so often, reread your past intentions to see if there is a theme or an area in which you could continue to improve.

ACCOUNTABILITY   Sharing your intentions with others provides a greater sense of accountability. You can share your intentions with friends, family members, or online through a variety of different outlets. A favorite is Intent.com, a wonderful resource started by Mallika Chopra, Deepak Chopra's daughter. She started Intent.com with the hope that community members would share their intents with others to gain support and keep them accountable. Share your intentions daily, weekly, or monthly for inspiration and encouragement.

✦ ✦ ✦

DEAL WITH DEMONS

Turn your wounds into wisdom.
—OPRAH WINFREY

OUR PAST IS made up of both positive and negative experiences. Although both are a natural part of life, when we struggle unsuccessfully to let go of the negative experiences—including past mistakes and unhealthy relationships that have caused hurt or disappointment—they quickly turn into our personal "demons," haunting us for years to come. These demons limit us in enjoying what life has to offer and keep us stuck. As a result, dealing with them is crucial to finding happiness, reducing stress, and moving forward with our dreams.

One of the biggest demons we typically fight is holding onto or regretting past mistakes. When we don't let go of the negativity of the past, we tend to let it define us today. Clinging to those experiences limits our future and our potential.

Other typical demons stem from our relationships. All of our relationships—including those with parents, siblings, friends, schoolmates, and, later in life, colleagues and significant others—influence how we behave and how we relate to others. If any of our relationships were (or are) unhealthy, abusive, or dysfunctional, the hurts and disappointments that resulted can take a toll on how we look at life, how we think about ourselves, and how we interact with others. They can create behaviors and fears that may not be rooted in the reality of today.

Accepting and letting go of past mistakes and unhealthy relationships enables us to learn valuable lessons so we can avoid making the same, or bigger, mistakes in the future. When we can overcome negative experiences and recover, we become more resilient to stress and adversity because we realize we can handle and move past hurt. Our demons can actually challenge us in a positive way, pushing us to make important changes and be a better version of ourselves, and to think in new and different ways. Dealing with demons makes us stronger and more capable to persevere through the ups and the downs.

✢ ✢ ✢

THE PATH TO CHANGE
LET GO OF NEGATIVITY FROM PAST EXPERIENCES

HOW WE DEAL with our demons can make or break our ability to be happy, to be the best possible version of ourselves, and to seize all that life has to offer. Some tips:

ACKNOWLEDGE AND IDENTIFY   Before you can deal with your demons, you have to acknowledge they are there. Most of us have them, and ignoring them or pretending that they don't exist leads to a state of denial, which can result in bigger problems. Acknowledge the past experiences that have negatively impacted you, and think about how they've shaped you. Use the questions in the "My Demons" section of the Demons Worksheet in Part III: Tools and Resources.

LEARN FROM YOUR DEMONS   Part of the reason it can be difficult to let go of the past is that we don't always think about what it has taught us.

Think about what you've learned from past negative experiences and write them down in the "Lessons Learned" section of the Demons Worksheet. When you start to resent or feel negatively toward the past, revisit the lessons learned and see them as invaluable blessings.

LET GO   The past is the past. What was, was. Let go of the negativity by doing the following:

Feel it   Allow yourself to feel the disappointment, hurt, or pain you feel. Don't hold back. If you want to cry, cry. If you want to be angry, be angry. Feeling the emotions is the first step to letting them go.

Be objective   Once you've felt what you needed to feel, move into an objective place that allows you to be more rational. Ask yourself what would make the emotion go away.

Forgive   Whether you need to forgive yourself or someone else, actively go through the process of forgiveness.

Look forward   Remember that failure, hurt, disappointment, and other negative experiences are all part of life. That being said, you have the power to not let the past hold you hostage. Redirect your thoughts to those that are more productive. See the future as a new chapter to re-create your reality and focus on what you want out of life. This will help you visualize positive outcomes, mobilizing you to make them a reality.

CREATE NEW ENERGY   Focusing on the past is limiting and keeps us in a place of immobility. More likely than not, you can work through a lot of your past so you can move forward and get beyond it. Use the "New Energy Creation" section of the Demons Worksheet to decide how you can let go of the negative feelings and use them to create a new, positive energy. This takes you out of a place of resentment and puts you in a more positive frame of mind and a place of proactive and rational thinking.

ABOLISH PAST LIMITATIONS   Embracing the possibility of negative outcomes should be seen as part of life and as part of growth. When we hold onto the past, it limits us because we (1) don't take risks or try new things out of fear of repeating past mistakes or making new ones, and (2) let it define us based on what we were or weren't able to do in the past. We tell ourselves "I can't," "I shouldn't," or "it won't work." Thinking "I can," "I should," or "I'll make it work" instead is much more productive and positive. Don't let the past define you. Think about how you *want* to be defined, and focus on making *that* your reality.

AVOID REPEATING HISTORY   Our demons often draw us to people or situations that bring out old comfortable habits. We are attracted to individuals with a similar history or who carry similar baggage. Unfortunately, this can keep us in an immobile and negative place, stuck in the same ruts, unhealthy behaviors, and toxic relationships. Be hyperaware of the circumstances you get into and avoid putting yourself in situations that let old, unhealthy habits resurface. Look for relationships that support healthier habits, and minimize those relationships that don't.

✣ ✣ ✣

TRAIN YOUR BRAIN

The brain is like a muscle. When it is in use we feel
very good. Understanding is joyous.

—CARL SAGAN

JUST AS PHYSICAL training does a body good, mental training does our
brain good. Recent research shows that brain fitness training, also known
as cognitive training, has a tremendous positive influence on brain
function. Cognitive training capitalizes on neuroplasticity and the idea
that cognitive function can be maintained or improved by putting your
mind through new and challenging experiences. In other words, training
your brain can boost brain function.

Brain-boosting exercises can significantly improve our working
memory (important for language comprehension, learning, and reasoning), our ability to pay attention and focus, and our ability to think faster
and remain mentally flexible.[1] Further, it can increase what is called
"fluid intelligence"—the ability to problem solve, regardless of former
acquired knowledge.[2]

Regularly training the brain also helps protect memory and can slow or
prevent age-related cognitive decline, Alzheimer's, and other forms of
dementia.[1] And the earlier you engage in these types of activities, the

better. One study found that people who engaged in cognitively challenging activities from childhood throughout adulthood had brains comparable to those who were fifty years younger, and they were less likely to develop the brain plaques associated with Alzheimer's disease.[3]

DID YOU KNOW?

In a study conducted by Lumos Labs, it was found that those who participated in a Web-based cognitive training program for twenty minutes a day for five weeks saw a significant improvement in their visual attention (20 percent) and their working memory (10 percent).[4]

Young minds can benefit from brain training as well. Studies show that cognitive training can help improve working memory in children, even positively affecting academic achievement.[5] Further, research has shown cognitive training can improve attention and organization and reduce symptoms in children with ADHD and other processing issues.[6]

THE PATH TO CHANGE
ENGAGE IN COGNITIVE TRAINING FOR TWENTY MINUTES EACH DAY

JUST TWENTY MINUTES of cognitive training each day can do a world of good. And the best part is, cognitive training can be fun! That said, although playing Sudoku or doing crossword puzzles each day can be fun or entertaining, these types of games do not really qualify as cognitive training. You may become better at those specific games but are not likely to see any real improvement in cognitive function. Instead, you need to engage your brain in novel, adaptive, and absorbing ways. Here's how:

HIT THE DIFFERENT CATEGORIES   Cognitive training should train your brain in four different areas:

Memory and recall Chess, cards, and crosswords

Attention and focus Reading comprehension, pattern memorization, and recognition

Cognition and problem solving Arithmetic and math; word problems

Speed and spatial reasoning Video games, Tetris, jigsaw puzzles, mazes, and navigation and orienteering

CROSS-TRAIN   Physical cross-training provides greater benefits to your physical health than doing the same form of exercise—such as running—every day. Mixing it up keeps your body on its toes, so to speak. This same concept holds true with your mind. You need to be challenged mentally in different ways to see greater benefits to your brain. To experience cognitive training, you'll want to rotate through the different categories above to keep your brain challenged by the unexpected. For instance, if you tend to play Sudoku every day, you'll want to rotate other games into the mix as well.

GO AGAINST THE CLOCK   Dr. Cynthia Green, author of _Brainpower Game Plan: Sharpen Your Memory, Improve Your Concentration, and Age-Proof Your Mind in Just 4 Weeks_, explains that timing yourself and working to beat the clock (or your best time for a game) is a great way to keep your brain challenged.

LEARN NEW GAMES   Be on the lookout for new games, and don't be afraid to try them. Search online for new books around brain fitness and other cognitive training programs; play new card games, and even indulge in new board games with your friends and family. Learning new rules and new formats of games will keep things fresh.

CHOOSE A PROGRAM   Although creating your own cognitive training program may seem ideal, the best way to engage in cognitive training is to sign up for a well-respected Web-based cognitive training program. Personally, I love Lumosity (www.lumosity.com), but there are plenty of other brain fitness programs out there. In choosing a Web-based program, however, you want to see certain criteria met. Here are some important questions to ask:

Is the program scientifically based? Ideally, neurologists, neuropsychologists, and scientists who understand the brain's structure and function should have developed the training program. Further, they should have research that backs up their program. As you know, companies are known for conducting their own research and touting claims that sound good, but if the research is designed, implemented, and reviewed internally, the programs may not be sound. Look for programs that have been researched and peer-reviewed. Some programs have even partnered with universities and medical institutions in their studies.

Is there real benefit? The point of brain training is that the skills you develop through the training should translate to real life. The cognitive training program you choose should be able to provide baseline assessments and post-training assessments separate from the training itself so you can see how you are improving. Further, the program should delineate which cognitive skills and what part of your brain you are training for each exercise.

Do exercises and games meet the following criteria?

❖ **THEY ARE NOVEL:** _Repetitively playing the same games each day will make you better at the game, but it won't necessarily improve your cognition. Any program you choose should have a wide variety of games, even within each area of training (for example, memory, flexibility, problem solving, and so on)._

❖ **THEY ARE TIMED:** _As Dr. Cynthia Green mentions, racing against a clock is important to training cognitive function. It helps your mind to work quickly, pay greater attention, and be more flexible._

✤ **THEY INCREASE IN DIFFICULTY:** *As you become faster and better at various games and exercises, you should advance to new and more difficult levels to stay challenged.*

MAKE IT SOCIAL   Playing games with others makes brain training more fun, and you'll reap the social benefits from it as well. If you enjoy card games, such as poker, get a group together for poker night once a week. Or book a weekly night of Scrabble with friends. If in-person games are difficult to coordinate, create weekly challenges with your friends to complete a crossword puzzle.

STEP AWAY FROM THE CALCULATOR   Calculators make it easy to avoid using your brain for even the simplest of math problems. Yet simple arithmetic can go a long way in keeping your brain on its toes. When you need to calculate the tip at a restaurant or need to know what a sale price is, try to figure it out in your head.

MEMORIZE A SONG OR POEM ONCE A WEEK   Even if you aren't interested in doing a poetry reading or singing in a band, memorizing songs and poems keeps your mind in memorizing mode. Try to memorize one per week to keep your brain working.

EXPAND YOUR VOCABULARY   Each day, learn a new word. Not only will you expand your vocabulary, but you will keep your memory sharp.

✤ ✤ ✤

ABOLISH
BRAIN KILLERS

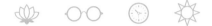

Garbage in, garbage out.
—**GEORGE FUECHSEL**

JUST AS THERE are many foods that promote brain health, there are also foods that can do the opposite. This week, you will focus on avoiding those foods that negatively impact cognitive function, cause mood swings, reduce energy, and add to stress.

Probably one of the top brain killing foods to avoid is added sugar. When we consume high amounts of sugar, it can negatively impact our mood and lead to an inevitable sugar crash. Consuming high amounts of sugar also has the power to interfere with our ability to learn. In a study out of UCLA, it was found that diets high in fructose (a form of sugar) over the long term alters your brain's ability to learn and remember information.[1]

And if sweets aren't your thing, you should know that foods high in sodium (salt) can have negative impacts on your brain as well. Studies show that diets high in salt impair your ability to think and may lead to dementia. A 2011 longitudinal study looked at 1,262 participants ranging in age from sixty-seven to eighty-four. Those who consumed the highest amounts of sodium showed declining scores on cognitive function tests over a three-year period, compared with those with the lowest salt intake.[2]

Another type of food that damages your brain is trans fats, often found in fried food, fast food, and junk food. Trans fats have been shown to negatively impact memory, attention, language skills, and processing speed, and can actually shrink the volume of your brain—a typical hallmark of Alzheimer's disease. In a study out of Oregon Health and Science University, blood samples and MRI scans were taken of 104 seniors. They found that those participants with the highest levels of trans fats in their blood also had smaller brains.[3]

Finally, many processed foods that contain artificial ingredients—including artificial sweeteners, additives, chemicals, dyes, and preservatives—should be avoided as well. More and more research shows that these ingredients negatively impact behavior and cognitive function and are linked to degenerative diseases, including Alzheimer's disease.[4]

✤ ✤ ✤

THE PATH TO CHANGE
AVOID FOODS THAT ARE HARMFUL TO BRAIN HEALTH

IF CUTTING OUT these foods seems like a difficult task, focus on making small shifts to your diet with these tips over time. Also, remember the less you eat these foods, the easier it will be to avoid them. We become less addicted as we reduce our intake.

AVOID PROCESSED FOODS Processed foods aren't found in nature on their own. Instead, they've been created through some type of manufacturing process. Everything from bread to frozen dinners to canned soup is processed food. As mentioned, processed foods tend to contain artificial ingredients, chemicals, and other additives. They also tend to contain added sugar, added salt and/or sodium, and, yes, trans fats, all of which are on the "avoid" list. So the easiest way to avoid brain-killing foods is to avoid foods that are processed. Whenever possible, choose fresh, whole foods.

KNOW THE SUGARY CULPRITS   Typical foods high in sugar include candy, soft drinks, energy drinks, syrup, jelly, protein bars, nutrition bars, cookies, and other baked goods. Also, it pays to know that added sugar comes in many forms. There are many aliases, but some of the more well known include brown sugar, brown rice syrup (or sugar), cane sugar, corn syrup, dextrose, fructose, high-fructose corn syrup, honey, molasses, and sucrose.

GET YOUR SWEET FIX   Whenever you want a sweet fix, choose foods that are naturally sweet, such as whole fruit. Natural sugar found in whole fruit isn't of concern. You can even use fruit to sweeten foods instead of sugar. For instance, use whole fruit in your smoothie instead of juice, honey, or sugar. You'll not only get the sweet taste, but you'll get the fiber as well, which will stabilize blood sugar and energy levels. And although artificial sweeteners may have fewer calories, they can be just as detrimental to your health and brain as sugar. Avoid these at all costs.

STAY HYDRATED   Lack of hydration can cause false hunger and feed into sugar cravings. If you are craving something sweet, try drinking a big glass of water. You may find that the water staves off the craving.

LOW-SUGAR BAKING   Sugar is a huge part of baking. That said, many recipes will taste just as good if you cut out 25 to 33 percent of the sugar. If a recipe calls for one cup of sugar, try using three-quarters of a cup and see how it tastes. Also, make use of sweeter spices, such as cinnamon, ginger, and nutmeg, to get a sweeter flavor without the harmful effects.

KNOW THE SALTY CULPRITS   Sodium is found in so many foods. Typical foods high in sodium are canned, prepackaged, and processed foods, including sauces, condiments, canned soups, snacks, and frozen foods, as well as cured meats and cold cuts. Sodium comes in many forms, including MSG, baking soda, baking powder, disodium phosphate, sodium alginate, and sodium nitrate.

15 PERCENT SODIUM OR LESS   Minimize your intake of the high-sodium foods just mentioned, and choose those labeled as low in sodium or that represent 15 percent of your total daily intake. Also, try to cut out premixed or prepared foods such as sauces, frozen pizzas, frozen dinners, and frozen foods in general, as they all tend to be high in sodium.

COOK WITH LESS SALT   You have the most control when you cook your own food. Experiment with spices other than salt. Garlic, pepper, curry, paprika, onion, oregano, parsley, cumin, thyme, rosemary, and many other spices give food wonderful flavor. The more a food is cooked, the more salt is diluted, so when you do choose to use salt, add it at the very end, as you will need much less.

AVOID TRANS FATS   In short, the best way to avoid trans fats is to avoid fast food and fried foods. Many processed, packaged foods contain trans fats, too, but because of the rise in awareness of these unhealthy fats, many companies have removed them from their products. The best practice, once again, is to opt for whole, fresh foods whenever possible.

✥ ✥ ✥

HAVE A
GENEROUS SPIRIT

What we have done for ourselves alone dies with us;
what we have done for others and the world remains
and is immortal.

— ALBERT PIKE

A GENEROUS SPIRIT IS a beautiful quality to have, and it is also good for your health, physically and mentally. Giving your time, energy, or money has the power to increase happiness and reduce risk of depression, decrease stress, and strengthen your relationships.

As it turns out, we are biologically wired to feel happier from having a generous spirit. When we give, our altruism activates regions in the brain associated with pleasure, social connection, and trust.[1] Acts of kindness have also been associated with a release of endorphins (hormones responsible for happiness) in the brain. These biological responses produce what has been termed a "helper's high," a euphoric feeling of calm and happiness.[2]

When we are generous, we also experience reduced stress. When we give of ourselves, our attention is drawn to the needs of others, so we are less focused on our own stress and problems. And exhibiting generosity has been shown to lower blood pressure as well as levels of cortisol, a stress hormone. Individuals who give social support also tend to exhibit greater self-efficacy and self-esteem and less depression.[3, 4]

Generosity toward others makes us less likely to think negatively about ourselves. Our generous nature helps us to be more sensitive to ourselves—silencing our inner critic and boosting self-confidence in the process. Whether we lend an ear to a friend having problems, give some guidance to a colleague, or take time to volunteer, we naturally increase our sense of purpose and self-worth, and we feel more fulfilled as a result.

GENEROSITY MAKES FOR A HAPPY MARRIAGE

According to a 2011 report from the National Marriage Project, generosity is a key factor in having a happy marriage. When partners give "good things freely and abundantly," meaning anything from showing affection to forgiveness to making their spouse a cup of coffee in the morning, it really adds up to something meaningful. Husbands and wives who score high on the generosity scale—in terms of both giving and receiving in a spirit of generosity—are at least 32 percent more likely to report that they are "very happy" in their marriages and less prone to divorce.[5]

When we demonstrate an open and generous heart, we attract others more easily. Even more important, we lay the foundation for stronger, more rewarding relationships. When we give to others, they are more likely to give back, and these exchanges between people encourage trust, cooperation, respect, and other positive feelings that strengthen ties. When we give, we see others more positively, which starts a beautiful cycle of positivity. In Sonja Lyubomirsky's book *The How of Happiness*, she explains, "Being kind and generous leads you to perceive others more positively and more charitably . . . and fosters a heightened sense of interdependence and cooperation in your social community."[6]

✤ ✤ ✤

THE PATH TO CHANGE
BE *MORE* GENEROUS

A GENEROUS SPIRIT IS one that is compassionate, helpful, and loving. Generosity comes from the heart, but is best demonstrated through our actions. Cultivate a generous spirit with some of the following ideas:

REMEMBER WHEN   As it turns out, thinking about the times when you were generous in the past (rather than times when you received help) can motivate you to be generous today.[7] Take a moment to remember times you displayed generosity, and use the Generosity Worksheet to describe what you did, how it helped others, and how you felt about the experience.

START AT HOME   Many people in our lives can use our warmth, compassion, and generosity. Pay attention to the people closest to you and look for opportunities to be helpful. Maybe you have an older family member who could use some help fixing things around the house. Maybe a nephew or niece could use your help with a science project. Or maybe your neighbor had surgery and could use a little extra help with grocery shopping and other errands. When you look for opportunities to be generous, you'll find ways to show your love and helpfulness every day.

BE PROACTIVE   The best way to show love and generosity is through your actions. Although telling someone you support them, love them, or are there for them is a great first step, find ways to *show* them you mean it. If you think someone could use your help, but they are too proud, shy, or uncomfortable to ask, take the initiative to find something to do that will be helpful.

SURROUND YOURSELF   The more time we spend with certain types of people, the more we are inclined to be like them. Generosity as a characteristic is extremely contagious. Surround yourselves with generous, loving people, and their warm nature will have a profound effect.

VOLUNTEER WITH PASSION   If you have the time (and most of us do), find ways to give some of it to volunteerism. Whether you choose to donate time to the local soup kitchen, go on a volunteer vacation, or become a "big sibling" for the local Big Brothers Big Sisters chapter in your area, choose something for which you have passion. When you give your time to something you care about, you'll not only feel good from the act of giving itself, but you'll also feel good about contributing to a cause that has significance to you.

ACCEPT GENEROSITY   Many of us feel comfortable giving but don't always feel comfortable being on the receiving end of other people's generosity. Accepting generosity from others, however, is just as important. When you feel yourself resistant to the help or generosity of others, remind yourself of how it makes you feel when you help someone, and remember that others feel the same when they help you! Be open to the generosity of others, and allow them to give you the support or help you need, when you need it.

✢ ✢ ✢

FOURTH QUARTER CHECKLIST

WEEKLY CHANGES	IN ACTION?
Week 1: Put Pen to Paper	☐
Week 2: Let the Music Play	☐
Week 3: Show Your Pearly Whites	☐
Week 4: Be a Goal Setter	☐
Week 5: Make Lists	☐
Week 6: Be a Mono-Tasker	☐
Week 7: Forget the Joneses	☐
Week 8: Meditate	☐
Week 9: Kick Indecision	☐
Week 10: Sip Green Tea	☐
Week 11: See the Best in Others	☐
Week 12: Read for Pleasure	☐
Week 13: Give Me a Break	☐
Week 14: Silence Your Inner Critic	☐
Week 15: Go Beyond Your Comfort Zone	☐
Week 16: Get Moving	☐
Week 17: Give Thanks	☐
Week 18: Place Value on Doing	☐
Week 19: Seek Silence	☐
Week 20: Speak Up	☐
Week 21: Put Time in a Box	☐
Week 22: Eat Good Fats	☐
Week 23: Open Your Mind	☐
Week 24: Sleep	☐
Week 25: Give Yourself a Time-Out	☐
Week 26: Be a Lifelong Learner	☐

Week 27: Minimize Screen Time ☐

Week 28: Reward Yourself ☐

Week 29: Say Yes to New Experiences ☐

Week 30: Get a Rubdown ☐

Week 31: Be Confident ☐

Week 32: Cultivate Creativity ☐

Week 33: Eat Brain-Boosting Fruits
and Vegetables ☐

Week 34: Go Alfresco ☐

Week 35: Skip the Small Talk ☐

Week 36: Send Out an S.O.S. ☐

Week 37: Get Out of Town ☐

Week 38: Take a Whiff ☐

Week 39: Face Fears ☐

Week 40: Practice De-Stressing Rituals ☐

Week 41: Reach Out and Touch
Someone ☐

Week 42: Be Hands-On ☐

Week 43: Be a Guru ☐

Week 44: Streamline Your Space ☐

Week 45: Build Close Relationships ☐

Week 46: Schedule To-Dos ☐

Week 47: Play ☐

Week 48: Set Intentions ☐

Week 49: Deal with Demons ☐

Week 50: Train Your Brain ☐

Week 51: Abolish Brain Killers ☐

Week 52: Have a Generous Spirit ☐

PART III

TOOLS AND RESOURCES

AS YOU NAVIGATE the small changes outlined throughout the book, use these tools and resources to help you through the program. Feel free to photocopy and paste them into your journal, write on them directly, or use them as guides to create your own assessments and worksheets.

If you would like to download these in a PDF format, please visit www.chroniclebooks.com/52SmallChangesfortheMind. This is your journey; feel free to customize the process to be your own!

MUSIC AND MOOD ASSESSMENT

What types of music do you enjoy?

....

....

What types of music do you dislike?

....

....

Fill out this chart with the types of music that elicit the emotions listed in the table. Use the blank spaces for any emotions not listed that you'd like to add.

ELICITED EMOTION OR MOOD	TYPE OF MUSIC
Happy	
Energized	
Safe and Comfortable	
Calm and Relaxed	
Focused / Able to Concentrate	
Inspired	
Motivated	
Creative	
Productive	
Excited	
Sad / Melancholy	
Based on the types of music you listed, create playlists to match your desired mood.	

SMARTE GOAL WORKSHEET

Go through the following questions to ensure that your goal is SMARTE.

IS IT SPECIFIC?

- What do you want to accomplish?

....

....

- Why is the goal important?

....

....

- Who else do you need to accomplish the goal?

....

....

- Where will you achieve the goal?

....

....

- Which steps are necessary in order to accomplish the goal?

....

....

- Is it measurable? How will you measure the results?

....

....

IS IT ACTIONABLE?

- Can you take action to work toward this goal?

....

....

- Do you have the power to achieve it?

....

....

IS IT RELEVANT?

- Is this goal meaningful to you?

....

....

- Does it match your needs and values?

....

....

IS IT TIMELY?

- When do you want to accomplish this goal?

....

....

- What can be accomplished in a few days? Weeks? Months? A year?

....

....

IS IT EMOTIONALLY DRIVEN?

- Are you excited about this goal?

....

....

- Do you feel inspired and motivated to accomplish it?

....

....

- Can you keep your motivation level high all the way through to completion?

....

....

NEGATIVE SELF-TALK ASSESSMENT

What negative thoughts do you have about yourself?

....

Do you really believe these thoughts to be true?

....

How do these thoughts make you feel? How are these thoughts impacting your life right now?

....

....

Where do these thoughts come from? A critical parent? A parent with low self-esteem? Your experience in school? Your friends?

....

....

How can you shift your thinking so that these thoughts are more positive?

....

PROVIDE FIVE EXAMPLES OF:

• What you love about yourself

....

• Your strengths

....

• Your accomplishments

....

COMFORT ZONE ASSESSMENT

On a scale of 1 to 10, with 1 being the least invigorated and 10 being the most, evaluate how invigorated you feel in the following areas in your life.

Work/Career	1	2	3	4	5	6	7	8	9	10
Friendships	1	2	3	4	5	6	7	8	9	10
Family	1	2	3	4	5	6	7	8	9	10
Spouse/Significant Other	1	2	3	4	5	6	7	8	9	10
Hobbies	1	2	3	4	5	6	7	8	9	10
Fitness/Health	1	2	3	4	5	6	7	8	9	10
Other Interests	1	2	3	4	5	6	7	8	9	10

Using the following chart as a template, enter how you'd like to challenge yourself to improve the areas in the Comfort Zone Assessment where you scored a six (6) or less. Enter a target date of completion in the right-hand column.

CHALLENGES TO CONSIDER

AREA OF LIFE	CHALLENGE TO PURSUE	TARGET DATE
		/ /
		/ /
		/ /
		/ /
		/ /
		/ /

GRATITUDE JOURNAL TEMPLATE

For whom/what are you feeling grateful today?

....

....

....

....

....

Were you surprised? Did something happen? What emotions did you feel?
Share the story.

....

....

....

....

....

How would life be different without this person, experience, thing for which
you're grateful?

....

....

....

....

....

NOISE INVENTORY WORKSHEET

Use the following chart to pinpoint where and when noise levels are at their peak in your environment. If noise levels are too high, consider what you can do to improve the situation.

TIME OF DAY	5 a.m.–8 a.m.

NOISE LEVEL IN YOUR ENVIRONMENT:

HOW DOES THIS NOISE LEVEL MAKE YOU FEEL?

WHAT CAN YOU DO TO POSITIVELY ALTER THE NOISE LEVEL?

TIME OF DAY	8 a.m.–Noon

NOISE LEVEL IN YOUR ENVIRONMENT:

HOW DOES THIS NOISE LEVEL MAKE YOU FEEL?

WHAT CAN YOU DO TO POSITIVELY ALTER THE NOISE LEVEL?

TIME OF DAY	Noon–3 p.m.

NOISE LEVEL IN YOUR ENVIRONMENT:

HOW DOES THIS NOISE LEVEL MAKE YOU FEEL?

WHAT CAN YOU DO TO POSITIVELY ALTER THE NOISE LEVEL?

TIME OF DAY   3 p.m. – 6 p.m.

NOISE LEVEL IN YOUR ENVIRONMENT:

HOW DOES THIS NOISE LEVEL MAKE YOU FEEL?

WHAT CAN YOU DO TO POSITIVELY ALTER THE NOISE LEVEL?

TIME OF DAY   6 p.m. – 10 p.m.

NOISE LEVEL IN YOUR ENVIRONMENT:

HOW DOES THIS NOISE LEVEL MAKE YOU FEEL?

WHAT CAN YOU DO TO POSITIVELY ALTER THE NOISE LEVEL?

TIME OF DAY   10 p.m. through the night

NOISE LEVEL IN YOUR ENVIRONMENT:

HOW DOES THIS NOISE LEVEL MAKE YOU FEEL?

WHAT CAN YOU DO TO POSITIVELY ALTER THE NOISE LEVEL?

SPEAK UP ASSESSMENT

When do you feel most comfortable speaking your mind?

....

....

When do you struggle to speak your mind?

....

....

What do you believe causes you to remain silent when voicing your feelings, thoughts, or opinions, when voicing them might benefit you?

....

....

What would be the best-case scenario as a result of your expressing yourself?

....

....

What would be the worst-case scenario from expressing yourself?

....

....

What could you do to rectify the worst-case scenario?

....

....

OPEN-MINDEDNESS ASSESSMENT

What are you most inclined to have a strong opinion about?

Do you know of any judgments or prejudices you hold?

Where do these judgments come from? Are they based on past experiences, upbringing, or something you've read or heard?

Do you believe these judgments to be 100 percent true or accurate?

For each device listed, log how much screen time you spend each day. Log the number of hours specific to work tasks in the first column and for personal use in the second column. Tally up the hours spent on each device, as well as the total amount of hours you spend on all screens per day. Set a goal of how much screen time you'd like to cut out of your week. Write these numbers in the right-hand column, "Goal."

TECHNOLOGY TYPE	HOURS PER DAY		TOTAL	GOAL
	WORK-RELATED	PERSONAL		
Television / Movies				
Video Games				
Television Screen Total:				
Internet				
Email				
IM/Chat				
Any Software/Application				
Computer Video				
Computer Screen Total:				
Mobile Internet				
Mobile Text/Messaging				
Mobile Video				
GPS Navigation				
Tablet				
eReaders				
Mobile Screen Total:				
Cinema				
Other				
Other Total:				
MEDIA TOTAL:				

CELEBRATE AND REWARD WORKSHEET

List five major accomplishments of which you are proud.

....

....

....

....

....

What did you do to accomplish each of these things?

....

....

....

....

....

What three words describe how you feel as a result of these accomplishments?

....

....

....

....

....

SELF-CONFIDENCE WORKSHEET

WHAT ARE YOUR STRENGTHS?

- What are you good at that doesn't require very much effort?

....

....

....

- What do you do better than most other people?

....

....

....

- When do you feel like you're in a "zone" of productivity, accomplishment, success, and happiness all at once?

....

....

....

WHAT ARE YOUR ACCOMPLISHMENTS?

- What accomplishments are you most proud of and why?

....

....

....

- What obstacles did you overcome during the process?

....

....

....

WHAT ARE YOUR MOST POSITIVE CHARACTERISTICS?

- What makes you special?

  ....

  ....

  ....

- What do people know they can count on about you?

  ....

  ....

  ....

- What do your friends, colleagues, and family think about you?

  ....

  ....

  ....

FEAR WORKSHEET

PAST FEARS

- What fears did you deal with in the past?

  ....

  ....

  ....

- How did they make you feel? What were you most afraid of?

  ....

  ....

  ....

- Were the fears based in reality? What caused them?

  ....

  ....

  ....

- What did you do or not do, and what was the result?

  ....

  ....

  ....

- If no action was taken, how did the fear hold you back? If action was taken, what were the benefits?

  ....

  ....

  ....

CURRENT FEARS

- What past fears do you still face today?

  ....

  ....

  ....

- What new fears have developed?

  ....

  ....

  ....

- Are these fears based in reality? What is causing them?

  ....

  ....

  ....

- What control do you have over these situations, and what can you do?

  ....

  ....

  ....

PLAY ASSESSMENT

What were your favorite activities as a child? What could you do for countless hours?

What did those activities make you feel?

How did those activities make you feel?

What can you do today that would elicit some of those same feelings?

What activities do you enjoy alone?

What activities make you lose your sense of time passing?

What activities do you enjoy with others?

A WEEK OF RESEARCH

Using the following chart, write down the activities you do over the course of the week and rate how much fun they are. In the right-hand column, assess whether you want to do more or less of the activity.

ACTIVITY	FUN (ON A SCALE OF 1 TO 10)										MORE OR LESS?
	1	2	3	4	5	6	7	8	9	10	
	1	2	3	4	5	6	7	8	9	10	
	1	2	3	4	5	6	7	8	9	10	
	1	2	3	4	5	6	7	8	9	10	
	1	2	3	4	5	6	7	8	9	10	
	1	2	3	4	5	6	7	8	9	10	
	1	2	3	4	5	6	7	8	9	10	
	1	2	3	4	5	6	7	8	9	10	
	1	2	3	4	5	6	7	8	9	10	
	1	2	3	4	5	6	7	8	9	10	

INTENTION JOURNAL TEMPLATE

TODAY'S INTENTION:

....

....

....

....

....

REFLECTIONS ON THE DAY'S INTENTION:

• Were you successful?

....

....

....

....

....

• What could you have done differently?

....

....

....

....

....

DEMONS WORKSHEET

YOUR DEMONS

- What past mistakes still upset you?

....

....

....

- What relationships caused (or still cause) you pain or hurt?

....

....

....

- What are you disappointed about?

....

....

....

- What regrets do you have?

....

....

....

LESSONS LEARNED

- What lessons did you learn from each of these?

....

....

....

NEW ENERGY CREATION

- What positives can you take away from your negative experiences?

....

....

....

- How can you apply lessons learned to create a new and more positive energy for the future?

....

....

....

- What in your life has gone well, and how can you apply that to the future?

....

....

....

GENEROSITY WORKSHEET

Describe a time you know you were generous.

....

....

....

....

What did you do?

....

....

....

....

How did it help others?

....

....

....

....

How did it make you feel?

....

....

....

....

NOTES

Week 1

1. Maria Christine Graf et al., "Written Emotional Disclosure: A Controlled Study of the Benefits of Expressive Writing Homework in Outpatient Psychotherapy," *Psychotherapy Research* 18, no. 4 (2008): 389–399, doi:10.1080/10503300701691664.

Week 2

1. John Noble Wilford, "Flute's Revised Age Dates the Sound of Music Earlier," *New York Times*, May 29, 2012, accessed July 12, 2012, http://www.nytimes.com/2012/05/29/science/oldest-musical-instruments-are-even-older-than-first-thought.html.

2. David B. Chamberlain, "Prenatal Stimulation: Experimental Results," *Birth Psychology*, accessed June 20, 2012, http://birthpsychology.com/free-article/prenatal-stimulation-experimental-results.

3. F. Rene Van de Carr and Marc Lehrer, "Enhancing Early Speech, Parental Bonding, and Infant Physical Development Using Prenatal Intervention in a Standard Obstetrical Practice," *Pre- & Perinatal Psychology Journal* 1, no. 1 (1986): 20–30.

4. Robert E. Krout, "The Effects of Single-Session Music Therapy Interventions on the Observed and Self-Reported Levels of Pain Control, Physical Comfort, and Relaxation of Hospice Patients," *American Journal of Hospice and Palliative Care* 18 (2001): 383–390.

5. Russell E. Hilliard, "The Effects of Music Therapy on the Quality and Length of Life of People Diagnosed with Terminal Cancer," *Journal of Music Therapy* 40 (2003): 113–137.

Week 3

1. Tara L. Kraft and Sarah D. Pressman, "Grin and Bear It: The Influence of Manipulated Facial Expression on the Stress Response," *Psychological Science*

23, no. 11 (2012): 1372–1378. http://pss.sagepub.com/content/early/2012/09/23/0956797612445312.

2. Chris L. Kleinke et al., "Effects of Self-Generated Facial Expressions on Mood," *Journal of Personality and Social Psychology* 74 (1998): 272–279.

3. Michael B. Lewis and Patrick J. Bowler, "Botulinum Toxin Cosmetic Therapy Correlates with a More Positive Mood," *Journal of Cosmetic Dermatology* 8 (2009): 24–26.

4. Ron Gutman, "The Hidden Power of Smiling," TED2011, March 2011, http://www.ted.com/talks/ron_gutman_the_hidden_power_of_smiling.html.

Week 4

1. "Study Backs Up Strategies for Achieving Goals," http://www.dominican.edu/dominicannews/study-backs-up-strategies-for-achieving-goals.

Week 5

1. Nancy Kalish, "Health Lessons from Your To-Do List," *Prevention* 61, no. 7 (2009): 76–78.

2. David Allen, *Getting Things Done: The Art of Stress-Free Productivity* (New York: Penguin Books, 2002), 40–41.

Week 6

1. J. M. Watson and D. L. Strayer, "Supertaskers: Profiles in Extraordinary Multitasking Ability," *Psychonomic Bulletin and Review* 17, no. 4 (2010): 479–485, doi:10.3758/PBR.17.4.479.

2. Eyal Ophir et al., "Cognitive Control in Media Multitaskers," *Proceedings of the National Academy of Sciences* 106:37 (2009): 15583–15587.

3. Russell Poldrack, University of California—Los Angeles, "Multi-Tasking Adversely Affects Brain's Learning, UCLA Psychologists Report," *ScienceDaily*, accessed November 10, 2013, www.sciencedaily.com/releases/2006/07/060726083302.htm.

4. Robert D. Rogers and Stephen Monsell, "Depth of Processing and the Retention of Words in Episodic Memory," *Journal of Experimental Psychology: General* 124, no. 2 (1995): 207–231.

5. Joshua S. Rubinstein et al., "Executive Control of Cognitive Processes in Task Switching," *Journal of Experimental Psychology: Human Perception and Performance* 27, no. 4 (2001): 763–797.

6. Zheng Wang and John M. Tchernev, "The 'Myth' of Media Multitasking: Reciprocal Dynamics of Media Multitasking, Personal Needs, and Gratifications," *Journal of Communication* 62, no. 3 (2012): 493–513.

7. "What Is Distracted Driving?" http://www.distraction.gov/content/get-the-facts/facts-and-statistics.html.

Week 7

1. Erzo F.P. Luttmer, "Neighbors as Negatives: Relative Earnings and Well-Being," *Quarterly Journal of Economics* 120, no. 3 (2005): 963–1002.

Week 8

1. Britta K. Hölzel et al., "Mindfulness Practice Leads to Increases in Regional Brain Gray Matter Density," *Psychiatry Research: Neuroimaging* 191, no. 1 (2011): 36–43.

2. David Levy and Jacob Wobbrock, "The Effects of Mindfulness Meditation Training on Multitasking in a High-Stress Information Environment," *Proceedings of Graphics Interface* (2012): 45–52.

Week 9

1. Sheena S. Iyengar and Mark R. Lepper, "When Choice Is Demotivating: Can One Desire Too Much of a Good Thing?" *Journal of Personality and Social Psychology* 79, no. 6 (2000): 995–1006.

Week 10

1. Gang Hu, Siamak Bidel, et al., "Coffee and Tea Consumption and the Risk of Parkinson's Disease," *Movement Disorders* 22, no. 15 (2007): 2242–2248.

2. Y. Wang, M. Li, et al., "Green Tea epigallocatechin-3-gallate (EGCG) Promotes Neural Progenitor Cell Proliferation and Sonic Hedgehog Pathway Activation during Adult Hippocampal Neurogenesis," *Molecular Nutrition and Food Research* 56, no. 8 (2012): 1292–1303.

3. "New Treatments Prevent Brain Injury Hours After Stroke in Rats," University of California – San Francisco, accessed December 12, 2013, http://www.eurekalert.org/pub_releases/2006-12/uoc--ntp122806.php.

4. Shinichi Kuriyama et al., "Green Tea Consumption and Cognitive Function: A Cross-Sectional Study from the Tsurugaya Project," *American Journal of Clinical Nutrition* 83, no. 2 (2006): 355–361.

5. Shinichi Kuriyama et al., "Green Tea Consumption Is Associated with Lower Psychological Distress in a General Population: The Ohsaki Cohort 2006 Study," *American Journal of Clinical Nutrition* 90, no. 5 (2009): 1390–1396.

6. Niu Kaijun Niu et al., "Green Tea Consumption Is Associated with Depressive Symptoms in the Elderly," *American Journal of Clinical Nutrition* 90, no. 6 (2009): 1615–1622.

7. Anna Christina Nobre et al., "L-theanine, a Natural Constituent in Tea, and Its Effect on Mental State," *Asia Pacific Journal of Clinical Nutrition* 17, no. 1 (2008): 167–168.

8. Gail N. Owen et al., "The Combined Effects of L-theanine and Caffeine on Cognitive Performance and Mood," *Nutritional Neuroscience* 11, no. 4 (2008): 193–198.

9. Simon P. Kelly et al., "L-Theanine and Caffeine in Combination Affect Human Cognition as Evidenced by Oscillatory Alpha-Band Activity and Attention Task Performance 1–3," *Journal of Nutrition* 138, no. 8 (2008): 1572S–1577S.

10. Shinichi Kuriyama et al., "Green Tea Consumption and Cognitive Function: A Cross-Sectional Study from the Tsurugaya Project," *American Journal of Clinical Nutrition* 83, no. 2 (2006): 355–361.

11. David J. Weiss and Christopher R. Anderton, "Determination of Catechins in Matcha Green Tea by Micellar Electrokinetic Chromatography," *Journal of Chromatography A* 1011(1–2) (2003): 173–180.

Week 11

1. Paul Rozin and Edward B. Royzman, "Negativity Bias, Negativity Dominance, and Contagion," *Personality and Social Psychology Review* 5, no. 4 (2001): 296–320.

2. Robert Rosenthal and Lenore Jacobson, *Pygmalion in the Classroom: Teacher Expectation and Pupils' Intellectual Development* (New York: Irvington Publishers, 1992).

Week 12

1. Anne E. Cunningham and Keith E. Stanovich, "What Reading Does for the Mind," *Journal of Direct Instruction* 1, no. 2 (2001): 137–149.

2. "Reading 'Can Help Reduce Stress,'" *Telegraph*, accessed March 1, 2014, http://www.telegraph.co.uk/health/healthnews/5070874/Reading-can-help-reduce-stress.html.

Week 13

1. Atsunori Ariga and Alejandro Lleras, "Brief and Rare Mental 'Breaks' Keep You Focused: Deactivation and Reactivation of Task Goals Preempt Vigilance Decrements," *Cognition* 118, no. 3 (2011): 439–43, doi:10.1016/j.cognition.2010.12.007.

2. Rana Balci and Fereydoun Aghazadeh, "The Effect of Work-Rest Schedules and Type of Task on the Discomfort and Performance of VDT Users," *Ergonomics* 46, no. 5 (2003): 455–465.

3. Chuansi Gao et al., "The Effects of VDT Data Entry Work on Operators," *Ergonomics* 33, no. 7 (1990): 917–923.

4. Linda Mclean et al., "Computer Terminal Work and the Benefit of Micro-breaks," *Applied Ergonomics* 32, no. 3 (2001): 225–237.

5. Robert A. Henning et al., "Frequent Short Rest Breaks from Computer Work: Effects on Productivity and Well-Being at Two Field Sites," *Ergonomics* 40, no. 1 (1997): 78–91.

Week 14

1. Erik J. Giltay et al., "Dispositional Optimism and the Risk of Depressive Symptoms during 15 Years of Follow-Up: The Zutphen Elderly Study," *Journal of Affective Disorders* 91 (2006): 45.

2. Ibid.

3. Ciro Conversano et al., "Optimism and Its Impact on Mental and Physical Well-Being," *Clinical Practice and Epidemiology in Mental Health* 6 (2010) 25–29, doi:10.2174/1745017901006010025.

Week 15

1. George E. Vaillant, *Triumphs of Experience: The Men of the Harvard Grant Study* (Cambridge, MA: Belknap Press, 2012).

Week 16

1. S. S. Lennox et al., "The Effect of Exercise on Normal Mood," *Journal of Psychosomatic Research* 34, no. 6 (1990): 629–636.

2 Stewart G. Trost, "Active Education: Physical Education, Physical Activity and Academic Performance," *Active Living Research* (2007): 1–3.

3. Ibid.

4. Ibid.

5. Ana C. Pereira et al., "An in vivo Correlate of Exercise-Induced Neurogenesis in the Adult Dentate Gyrus," *Proceedings of the National Academy of Sciences USA* 104 (2007): 5638–5643.

6. Kathryn Reid et al., "Aerobic Exercise Improves Self-Reported Sleep and Quality of Life in Older Adults with Insomnia," *Sleep Medicine* 11, no. 9 (2010): 934–940.

Week 17

1. Monica Y. Bartlett and David DeSteno, "Gratitude and Prosocial Behavior: Helping When It Costs You," *Psychological Science* 17, no. 4 (2006): 319–325.

2. Alex M. Wood et al., "Gratitude and Well-Being: A Review and Theoretical Integration," *Clinical Psychology Review* 30, no. 7 (2010): 890–905.

3. Robert Emmons, *Thanks!: How Practicing Gratitude Can Make You Happier* (New York: Mariner Books; reprint edition 2008), 30.

4. Alex M. Wood et al., "Gratitude Influences Sleep through the Mechanism of Pre-Sleep Cognitions," *Journal of Psychosomatic Research* 66, no. 1 (2009): 43–48.

5. Sara Algoe et al., "It's the Little Things: Everyday Gratitude as a Booster Shot for Romantic Relationships," *Personal Relationships* 17 (2010): 217–233.

6. Robert Emmons and Michael McCullough, "Counting Blessings versus Burdens: An Experimental Investigation of Gratitude and Subjective Well-Being in Daily Life," *Journal of Personality and Social Psychology* 84, no. 2 (2003): 377–389.

Week 18

1. Leaf Van Boven and Thomas Gilovich, "To Do or to Have? That Is the Question," *Journal of Personality and Social Psychology* 85, no. 6 (2003): 1193–1202.

2. Angus Deaton and Daniel Kahneman, "High Income Improves Evaluation of Life but Not Emotional Well-Being," *Proceedings of the National Academy of Sciences of the United States of America* 107, no. 38 (2010): 16489–16493, doi:10.1073/pnas.1011492107.

3. Peter A. Caprariello and Harry T. Reis, "To Do, to Have, or to Share? Valuing Experiences over Material Possessions Depends on the Involvement of Others," *Journal of Personality and Social Psychology* 104, no. 2 (2013): 199–215.

4. Thomas DeLeire and Ariel Kalil, "Does Consumption Buy Happiness? Evidence from the United States," *International Review of Economics* 57, no. 2 (2010): 163–176.

Week 19

1. Staffan Hygge et al., "The Munich Airport Noise Study: Cognitive Effects on Children from Before to After the Change Over of Airports," in *Proceedings of Inter-Noise '96 (Book 5)* (Liverpool, UK: Institute of Acoustics, 1996), 2189–2192.

2. V. J. Konenci, "The Mediation of Aggressive Behavior: Arousal Level versus Anger and Cognitive Labeling," *Journal of Personality and Social Psychology* 32 (1975): 706–712.

3. Sheldon Cohen, "Apartment Noise, Auditory Discrimination, and Reading Ability in Children," *Journal of Experimental Social Psychology* 9 (1973): 407–422.

4. Arline Bronzaft and Dennis McCarthy, "The Effects of Elevated Train Noise on Reading Ability," *Environmental Behavior* 7 (1975): 517–527.

5. "Noise-Induced Hearing Loss," National Institute of Deafness and Other Communication Disorders, NIH Pub. No. 13-4233, October 2013, http://www .nidcd.nih.gov/health/hearing/pages/noise.aspx.

Week 20

1. Marcus Mund and Kristin Mitte, "The Costs of Repression: A Meta-Analysis on the Relation between Repressive Coping and Somatic Diseases," *Health Psychology* 31, no. 5 (2012): 640–649, doi:10.1037/a0026257.

2. Christopher F. Karpowitz et al., "Gender Inequality in Deliberative Participation," *American Political Science Review* 106 (2012): 533–547, doi:10.1017/ S0003055412000329.

Week 22

1. Sandra Kalmijn et al., "Dietary Intake of Fatty Acids and Fish in Relation to Cognitive Performance at Middle Age," *Neurology* 62, no. 2 (2004): 275–280, doi:10.1212/01.WNL.0000103860.75218.A5.

2. W. L. Chung et al., "Fish Oil Supplementation of Control and (n-3) Fatty Acid-Deficient Male Rats Enhances Reference and Working Memory Performance and Increases Brain Regional Docosahexaenoic Acid Levels," *Journal of Nutrition* 138, no. 6 (2008): 1165–1171.

3. Alec Coppen and Christina Bolander-Gouaille, "Treatment of Depression: Time to Consider Folic Acid and Vitamin B12," *Journal of Psychopharmacology* 19, no. 1 (2005): 59–65.

4. Tyler Graham and Drew Ramsey, *The Happiness Diet: A Nutritional Prescription for a Sharp Brain, Balanced Mood, and Lean, Energized Body* (New York: Rodale, 2011), 113.

5. Peter Pribis et al., "Effects of Walnut Consumption on Cognitive Performance in Young Adults," *British Journal of Nutrition* 19 (2011): 1–9.

6. "Diet of Walnuts, Blueberries Found to Improve Cognition; May Help Maintain Brain Function and Treat Brain Disorders," *Society for Neuroscience*, modified November 5, 2007, http://www.sfn.org/Press-Room/News-Release-Archives/2007/DIET-OF-WALNUTS.

7. Olivia L. Okereke et al., "Dietary Fat Types and 4-Year Cognitive Change in Community-Dwelling Older Women," *Annals of Neurology* 72 (2012): 124–134, doi:10.1002/ana.23593.

8. University of Granada. "Vitamin B: Choline Intake Improves Memory and Attention-Holding Capacity, Experts Say," ScienceDaily. Accessed June 8, 2014, www.sciencedaily.com/releases/2013/07/130711103239.htm.

9. Poly Coreyann et al., "The Relation of Dietary Choline to Cognitive Performance and White-Matter Hyperintensity in the Framingham Offspring Cohort," *American Journal of Clinical Nutrition* 94, no. 6 (2011): 1584–1591, doi:10.3945/ajcn.110.008938.

10. Mitch Kanter et al., "Exploring the Factors That Affect Blood Cholesterol and Heart Disease Risk: Is Dietary Cholesterol as Bad for You as History Leads Us to Believe?" *Advances in Nutrition* 3, no. 5 (2012): 711–717, doi:10.3945/an.111.001321.

Week 24

1. Katharine Busby and R. T. Pivik, "Sleep Patterns in Children of Superior Intelligence," *Journal of Child Psychology and Psychiatry* 24 (1983): 587–600.

2. "Sleep Disorders and Sleep Deprivation: An Unmet Public Health Problem," Institute of Medicine, accessed May 12, 2014, http://www.ncbi.nlm.nih.gov/books/NBK19961.

3. Francesco P. Cappuccio et al., "Sleep Duration Predicts Cardiovascular Outcomes: A Systematic Review and Meta-Analysis of Prospective Studies," *European Heart Journal* 32, no. 12 (2011): 1484–1492, doi:10.1093/eurheartj/ehr007.

4. "How Much Sleep Do We Really Need?" National Sleep Foundation, accessed March 15, 2014, http://www.sleepfoundation.org/article/how-sleep-works/how-much-sleep-do-we-really-need.

5. S. H. Onen et al., "Prevention and Treatment of Sleep Disorders through Regulation of Sleeping Habits," *Presse Medicale* 23, no. 10 (1994): 485–489.

6. Kathryn J. Reid et al., "Aerobic Exercise Improves Self-Reported Sleep and Quality of Life in Older Adults with Insomnia," *Sleep Medicine* 11, no. 9 (2010): 934–940, doi:10.1016/j.sleep.2010.04.014.

Week 26

1. Pasko Rakic, "Neurogenesis in Adult Primate Neocortex: An Evaluation of the Evidence," *Nature Reviews Neuroscience* 3, no. 1 (2002): 65–71.

2. Peter S. Eriksson et al., "Neurogenesis in the Adult Human Hippocampus," *Nature Medicine* 4 (1998): 1313–1317.

3. Eleanor A. Maguire, "London Taxi Drivers and Bus Drivers: A Structural MRI and Neuropsychological Analysis," *Hippocampus* 16 (2006): 1091–1101.

Week 27

1. Edward L. Swing et al., "Television and Video Game Exposure and the Development of Attention Problems," *Pediatrics* 126, no. 2 (2010): 214–221, doi:10.1542/peds.2009-1508.

2. Dimitri A. Christakis et al., "Early Television Exposure and Subsequent Attentional Problems in Children," *Pediatrics* 113 (2004): 708.

3. Sarah Thomeé, "ICT Use and Mental Health in Young Adults: Effects of Computer and Mobile Phone Use on Stress, Sleep Disturbances, and Symptoms of Depression" (Ph.D. diss., University of Gothenberg, 2012).

4. John P. Robinson and Steven Martin, "What Do Happy People Do?" *Social Indicators Research* 89, no. 3 (2008): 565–571.

5. "Digital Set to Surpass TV in Time Spent with US Media," eMarketer, accessed April 12, 2014, http://www.emarketer.com/Article/Digital-Set-Surpass-TV-Time-Spent-with-US-Media/1010096.

6. "Screens to the nth: What Are People Doing and Why?", IAB, accessed April 5, 2014, http://www.iab.net/media/file/Simultaneous-screen-IAB-Innovation-Day-v19.pdf.

Week 28

1. Josh Bersin, "How the Trust Hormone Drives Business Performance," *Forbes*, April 30, 2012, http://www.forbes.com/sites/joshbersin/2012/04/30/how-the-trust-molecule-drives-business-performance.

2. "Motivating People: Getting Beyond Money," June 2009 McKinsey Global Survey, accessed April 5, 2014, http://www.mckinsey.com/insights/organization/motivating_people_getting_beyond_money.

3. Ibid.

1. Tiffany Field et al., "Pregnant Women Benefit from Massage Therapy," *Journal of Psychosomatic Obstetrics and Gynecology* 20 (1999): 31–38.

2. Tiffany Field et al., "Cortisol Decreases and Serotonin and Dopamine Increase Following Massage Therapy," *International Journal of Neuroscience* 115, no. 10 (2005): 1397–1413.

3. Melodee Harris et al., "The Effects of Slow-Stroke Back Massage on Minutes of Nighttime Sleep in Persons with Dementia and Sleep Disturbances in the Nursing Home: A Pilot Study," *Journal of Holistic Nursing* 30, no. 4 (2012): 255–263, doi:10.1177/0898010112455948.

4. Sheleigh Lawler and Linda D. Cameron, "A Randomized, Controlled Trial of Massage Therapy as a Treatment for Migraine," *Annals of Behavioral Medicine* 32, no. 1 (2006): 50–59.

5. Mark H. Rapaport et al., "A Preliminary Study of the Effects of Repeated Massage on Hypothalamic-Pituitary-Adrenal and Immune Function in Healthy Individuals: A Study of Mechanisms of Action and Dosage," *Journal of Alternative and Complementary Medicine* 18, no. 8 (2012): 789–797, doi:10.1089/acm.2011.0071.

6. Anne M. Jensen et al., "The Benefits of Giving a Massage on the Mental State of Massage Therapists: A Randomized, Controlled Trial," *Journal of Alternative and Complementary Medicine* 18, no. 12 (2012): 1142–6, doi:10.1089/acm.2011.0643.

7. Tiffany Field et al., "Elder Retired Volunteers Benefit from Giving Massage Therapy to Infants," *Journal of Applied Gerontology* 17 (1998): 229–239.

1. University of Melbourne, "Self-Confidence the Secret to Workplace Advancement," ScienceDaily, accessed February 10, 2014, http://www.sciencedaily.com/releases/2012/10/121018103214.htm>.

2. Amy Cuddy, "Your Body Language Shapes Who You Are," TED Talk, accessed March 10, 2014, http://www.ted.com/talks/amy_cuddy_your_body_language_shapes_who_you_are.

Week 32

1. Heather L. Stuckey et al., "The Connection Between Art, Healing, and Public Health: A Review of Current Literature," *American Journal of Public Health* 100, no. 2 (2010): 254–263.

2. Daniel Monti et al., "A Randomized, Controlled Trial of Mindfulness-Based Art Therapy (MBAT) for Women with Cancer," *Psycho-Oncology* 15, no. 5 (2006): 363–373.

3. Denise M. Sloan et al., "Written Exposure as an Intervention for PTSD: A Randomised Clinical Trial with Motor Vehicle Accident Survivors," *Behaviour, Research & Therapy* 50 (2012): 627–635.

4. Susan H. McFadden and Anne D. Basting, "Healthy Aging Persons and Their Brains: Promoting Resilience through Creative Engagement," *Clinical Geriatric Medicine* 26, no. 1 (2010): 149–161.

Week 33

1. Elizabeth E. Devore et al., "Dietary Intakes of Berries and Flavonoids in Relation to Cognitive Decline," *Annals of Neurology* 72, no. 1 (2012): 135–143, doi:10.1002/ana.23594.

2. Paula C. Bickford et al., "Antioxidant-Rich Diets Improve Cerebellar Physiology and Motor Learning in Aged Rats," *Brain Research* 866, no. 1–2 (2000): 211–217, http://dx.doi.org/10.1016/S0006-8993(00)02280-0.

3. Radiological Society of North America, "Coffee Jump-Starts Short-Term Memory," ScienceDaily, accessed April 3, 2014, www.sciencedaily.com/releases/2005/12/051212091544.htm.

4. Boukje M. van Gelder et al., "Coffee Consumption Is Inversely Associated with Cognitive Decline in Elderly European Men: the FINE Study," *European Journal of Clinical Nutrition (Impact Factor: 2.76)* 61, no. 2 (2007): 226–232, doi:10.1038/sj.ejcn.1602495.

5. Tennille D. Presley et al., "Acute Effect of a High Nitrate Diet on Brain Perfusion in Older Adults," *Nitric Oxide* 24, no. 1 (2011): 34–42, doi:10.1016/j.niox.2010.10.002.

6. John P. Docherty et al., "A Double-Blind, Placebo-Controlled, Exploratory Trial of Chromium Picolinate in Atypical Depression: Effect on Carbohydrate Craving," *Journal of Psychiatric* 11, no. 5 (2005): 302–314.

Week 34

1. "Questions about Your Community: Indoor Air," Environmental Protection Agency, accessed January 5, 2014, http://www.epa.gov/region1/communities/indoorair.html.

2. Darryl Eyles et al., "Vitamin D3 and Brain Development," *Neuroscience* 118, no. 3 (2003): 641–653.

3. Allen T. G. Lansdowne and Stephen C. Provost, "Vitamin D3 Enhances Mood in Healthy Subjects during Winter," *Psychopharmacology (Berl)* 135, no. 4 (1998): 319–323.

4. American Academy of Sleep Medicine, "Study Links Workplace Daylight Exposure to Sleep, Activity, and Quality of Life," *ScienceDaily*, accessed February 3, 2014, www.sciencedaily.com/releases/2013/06/130603114000.htm.

5. Michael F. Holick, "Vitamin D Deficiency," *New England Journal of Medicine* 357 (2007): 266–281, doi:10.1056/NEJMra070553.

6. Jane L. Harte and Georg H. Eifert, "The Effects of Running, Environment, and Attentional Focus on Athletes' Catecholamine and Cortisol Levels and Mood," *Psychophysiology* 32, no. 1 (1995): 49–54, doi:10.1111/j.1469-8986.1995.tb03405.x.

7. Bill Wolverton et al., "Interior Landscape Plants for Indoor Air Pollution Abatement," NASA/ALCA Final Report, Plants for Clean Air Council, Davidsonville, Maryland, 1989.

Week 35

1. Matthias R. Mehl et al., "Eavesdropping on Happiness: Well-Being Is Related to Having Less Small Talk and More Substantive Conversations," *Psychological Science* 21 (2010): 539–541.

Week 37

1. Heart + Mind Strategies, "American Vacation Opinions: Report on Key Findings" (2012).

2. "Expedia Vacation Deprivation Study 2012," *Expedia*, p. 53, accessed March 21, 2014, http://media.expedia.com/media/content/expus/graphics/other/pdf/Expedia-VacationDeprivation2012.pdf.

3. Colette Fabrigoule et al., "Social and Leisure Activities and Risk of Dementia: A Prospective Longitudinal Study," *Journal of the American Geriatrics Society* 43, no. 5 (1995): 485–490.

4. "Family Vacations Create Lasting Memories" explores the vacation habits of American families and how memories from family vacations are valued, captured, and shared. Harris Interactive conducted the online survey in December 2012 on behalf of the U.S. Travel Association. The survey included 2,531 adults and 1,130 youth ages eight to eighteen.

5. "Expedia Vacation Deprivation Study 2012," *Expedia*, accessed March 20, 2014, http://www.expedia.com/p/info-other/vacation_deprivation.htm.

Week 38

1. Amy Paturel, "What the Nose Knows," *Neurology Now* 3, no. 5 (2007): 42–43.

2. Shinichiro Haze et al., "Effects of Fragrance Inhalation on Sympathetic Activity in Normal Adults," *Japanese Journal of Pharmacology* 90, no. 3 (2002): 247–253.

3. Sioh Kim et al., "The Effect of Lavender Oil on Stress, Bispectral Index Values, and Needle Insertion Pain in Volunteers," *Journal of Alternative and Complementary Medicine* 17, no. 9 (2011): 823–826; Sun-Young Lee, "The Effect of Lavender Aromatherapy on Cognitive Function, Emotion, and Aggressive Behavior of Elderly with Dementia," *Taehan Kanho Hakhoe Chi* 35, no. 2 (2005, April): 303–312; George T. Lewith et al., "A Single-Blinded, Randomized Pilot Study Evaluating the Aroma of Lavandula Angustifolia as a Treatment for Mild Insomnia," *Journal of Alternative and Complementary Medicine* 11, no. 4 (2005, August): 631–637; Inn-Sook Lee and Gyung-Joo Lee, "Effects of Lavender Aromatherapy on Insomnia and Depression in Women College Students," *British Journal of Pharmacology* 128, no. 2 (1999, September): 380–384; Payam Sasannejad et al., "Lavender Essential Oil in the Treatment of Migraine Headache: A Placebo-Controlled Clinical Trial," *European Neurological Journal* 67, no. 5 (2012): 288–291.

4. Mark Moss et al., "Aromas of Rosemary and Lavender Essential Oils Differentially Affect Cognition and Mood in Healthy Adults," *International Journal of Neuroscience* 113, no. 1 (2003): 15–38.

Week 40

1. David Eilam et al., "Threat Detection: Behavioral Practices in Animals and Humans," *Neuroscience & Biobehavioral Reviews* 35, no. 4 (2011): 999, doi:10.1016/j.neubiorev.2010.08.002.

Week 41

1. Tiffany Field, "Preterm Infant Massage Therapy Research: A Review," *Infant Behavioral Development* 33, no. 2 (2010): 115–124, doi:10.1016/j.infbeh.2009.12.004.

2. James A. Coan et al., "Lending a Hand: Social Regulation of the Neural Response to Threat," *Psychological Science* 17, no. 12 (2006): 1032–1039.

3. Kathleen C. Light et al., "More Frequent Partner Hugs and Higher Oxytocin Levels Are Linked to Lower Blood Pressure and Heart Rate in Premenopausal Women," *Biological Psychology* 69, no. 1 (2005): 5–21.

4. Dacher Keltner, "Hands on Research: The Science of Touch," *The Greater Good*, September 29, 2010, http://greatergood.berkeley.edu/article/item/hands_on_research.

5. Eija Bergroth et al., "Respiratory Tract Illnesses During the First Year of Life: Effect of Dog and Cat Contacts," *Pediatrics* 130, no. 2 (2012): 211–220, doi:10.1542/peds.2011–2825.

6. Julia K. Vormbrock and John M. Grossberg, "Cardiovascular Effects of Human–Pet Dog Interactions," *Journal of Behavioral Medicine* 11, no. 5 (1988): 509–517.

Week 42

1. Kelly Lambert, *Lifting Depression: A Neuroscientist's Hands-On Approach to Activating Your Brain's Healing Power* (New York: Basic Books, 2008), 7, 33.

2. Ibid.

3. Christopher A. Lowry et al., "Identification of an Immune-Responsive Mesolimbocortical Serotonergic System: Potential Role in Regulation of Emotional Behavior," *Neuroscience* 146, no. 2 (2007): 756–772.

Week 43

1. Carolyn Schwartz et al., "Altruistic Social Interest Behaviors Are Associated with Better Mental Health," *Psychosomatic Medicine* 65, no. 5 (2003): 778–785, doi:10.1097/01.PSY.0000079378.39062.D4.

2. K. N. Rekha and M. P. Ganesh, "Do Mentors Learn by Mentoring Others?" *International Journal of Mentoring and Coaching in Education* 1, no. 3 (2012): 205–217.

3. Making a Difference: An Impact Study of Big Brothers Big Sisters—A Publication of Public/Private Ventures—September 2000.

Week 44

1. Stephanie A. McMains and Sabine Kastner, "Interactions of Top-Down and Bottom-Up Mechanisms in Human Visual Cortex," *Journal of Neuroscience* 31, no. 2 (2011): 587597, doi:10.1523/JNEUROSCI.3766-10.2011.

2. Mervin Blair et al., "The Role of Age and Inhibitory Efficiency in Working Memory Processing and Storage Components," *Quarterly Journal of Experimental Psychology* 64, no. 6 (2011): 1157–1172, doi:10.1080/17470218.2010.540670.

Week 45

1. Ryan E. Adams et al., "The Presence of a Best Friend Buffers the Effects of Negative Experiences," *Developmental Psychology* 47, no. 6 (2011): 1786–1791.

2. Karen A. Ertel et al., "Effects of Social Integration on Preserving Memory Function in a Nationally Representative US Elderly Population," *American Journal of Public Health* 98, no. 7 (2008): 1215–1220.

3. Bryan D. James et al., "Late-Life Social Activity and Cognitive Decline in Old Age," *Journal of the International Neuropsychological Society* 17, no. 6 (2011): 998–1005.

4. Julianne Holt-Lunstad et al., "Social Relationships and Mortality Risk: A Meta-Analytic Review," *PLoS Medicine* 7, no. 7 (2010): e1000316, doi:10.1371/journal.pmed.1000316.

5. Archana Singh and Nishi Misra, "Loneliness, Depression, and Sociability in Old Age," *Industrial Psychiatry Journal* 18, no. 1 (2009): 51–55.

Week 46

1. Marcus Austin, "Wasted time in meetings costs businesses £26 billion: The average employee wastes two hours and 39 minutes in meetings every week," *Techradar*, May 21, 2012, accessed September 15, 2014, http://www.techradar .com/us/news/world-of-tech/roundup/wasted-time-in-meetings-costs-businesses-26-billion-1081238.

2. "Opinion Matters," for Epson and the Centre for Economics and Business Research, May 2010.

Week 47

1. Stuart Brown, *Play: How It Shapes the Brain, Opens the Imagination, and Invigorates the Soul* (New York: Penguin, 2009).

Week 48

1. Alvaro Pascual-Leone et al., "The Plastic Human Brain Cortex," *Annual Review of Neuroscience* 28 (2005): 377–401.

2. Deepak Chopra, "5 Steps to Setting Powerful Intentions," http://www.chopra .com/ccl/5-steps-to-setting-powerful-intentions.

Week 50

1. Sherry L. Willis et al., "Long-term Effects of Cognitive Training on Everyday Functional Outcomes in Older Adults," *Journal of the American Medical Association* 296, no. 23 (2006): 2805–2814.

2. Susanne M. Jaeggi et al., "Improving Fluid Intelligence with Training on Working Memory," *Proceedings of the National Academy of Sciences of the United States of America* 105, no. 19 (2008): 6829–6833.

3. Susan M. Landau et al., "Association of Lifetime Cognitive Engagement and Low β-Amyloid Deposition," *Archives of Neurology* 69, no. 5 (2012): 623–629.

4. Joe Hardy et al., "Enhancing Visual Attention and Working Memory with a Web-Based Cognitive Training Program," *Mensa Research Journal* 42, no. 2 (2011): 13–20.

5. Adele Diamond and Kathleen Lee, "Interventions Shown to Aid Executive Function Development in Children 4 to 12 Years Old," *Science* 333, no. 6045 (2011): 959–964.

6. Steven J. Beck et al., "A Controlled Trial of Working Memory Training for Children and Adolescents with ADHD," *Journal of Clinical Child & Adolescent Psychology* 39, no. 6 (2010): 825–836.

Week 51

1. Rahul Agrawal and Fernando Gomez-Pinilla, "'Metabolic Syndrome' in the Brain: Deficiency in Omega-3 Fatty Acid Exacerbates Dysfunctions in Insulin Receptor Signalling and Cognition," *Journal of Physiology* 590, no. 10 (2012): 2485–99, doi:10.1113/jphysiol.2012.230078.

2. Alexandra J. Fiocco et al., "Sodium Intake and Physical Activity Impact Cognitive Maintenance in Older Adults: The NuAge Study," *Neurobiology of Aging* 33, no. 4 (2012): 829.e21–8, doi:10.1016/j.neurobiolaging.2011.07.004.

3. Gene L. Bowman et al., "Nutrient Biomarker Patterns, Cognitive Function, and MRI Measures of Brain Aging," *Neurology* 78, no. 4 (2012): 24–249, doi:10.1212/WNL.0b013e3182436598.

4. Russell L Blaylock, *Excitotoxins: The Taste That Kills* (Santa Fe: Health Press, 1997).

Week 52

1. Jorge Moll et al., "Human Fronto–Mesolimbic Networks Guide Decisions about Charitable Donation," *Proceedings of the National Academy of Sciences* 103, no. 42 (2006): 15623–15628, doi:10.1073/pnas.0604475103.

2. Allan Luks and Peggy Payne, *The Healing Power of Doing Good: The Health and Spiritual Benefits of Helping Others* (New York: iUniverse.com, 2001).

3. Rachel L. Piferi and Kathleen A. Lawler, "Social Support and Ambulatory Blood Pressure: An Examination of Both Receiving and Giving," *International Journal of Psychophysiology* 62 (2006): 328–336.

4. Elizabeth W. Dunn et al., "On the Costs of Self-Interested Economic Behavior: How Does Stinginess Get Under the Skin?" *Journal of Health Psychology* 15 (2010): 627–633, doi:10.1177/1359105309356366.

5. "The State of Our Unions: Marriage in America 2011," National Marriage Project and the Institute for American Values, accessed May 2, 2014, http://nationalmarriageproject.org/wp-content/uploads/2012/05/Union_2011.pdf.

6. Sonja Lyubomirsky, *The How of Happiness: A Scientific Approach to Getting the Life You Want* (New York: Penguin, 2008), 129.

7. Adam Grant and Jane Dutton, "Beneficiary or Benefactor: The Effects of Reflecting about Receiving versus Giving on Prosocial Behavior," *Psychological Science* 23, no. 9 (2012): 1033–1039.

ACKNOWLEDGMENTS

I WOULD LIKE TO express my sincere thanks to all of the individuals who have contributed to making *52 Small Changes for the Mind* possible.

Thank you to my agents, Meg Thompson and Sandy Hodgman, for their enthusiasm and excitement about this book and for finding it a perfect home. Thank you to the team at Chronicle Books for your time, dedication, and support; and for being with me every step of the way through editing, design, marketing, and publicity. To my editors Laura Lee Mattingly and Sara Golski, thank you for passionately working with me, and for your guidance and insight. Your commitment has been deeply appreciated. Kristi Hein, you brought levity and enjoyment to a rather tedious task. Kathie Gordon, your thoroughness is a godsend. And, Allison Weiner and Amanda Sim, your artistic creativity has been a joy. Yolanda Cazares and Steve Kim, thank you, too, for making the process feel so seamless. And, Stephanie Wong, I'm thrilled to have your marketing genius in my corner!

Finally, thank you to David and Alexander, my two greatest joys. And, thank you to Mom and Bill, for your constant support.

INDEX